Songs of the South African AIDS Crisis

Songs of the South African AIDS Crisis

Gavin Robert Walker

BLOOMSBURY ACADEMIC
NEW YORK • LONDON • OXFORD • NEW DELHI • SYDNEY

BLOOMSBURY ACADEMIC
Bloomsbury Publishing Inc, 1359 Broadway, New York, NY 10018, USA
Bloomsbury Publishing Plc, 50 Bedford Square, London, WC1B 3DP, UK
Bloomsbury Publishing Ireland, 29 Earlsfort Terrace, Dublin 2, D02 AY28, Ireland

BLOOMSBURY, BLOOMSBURY ACADEMIC and the Diana logo are trademarks of Bloomsbury Publishing Plc

First published in the United States of America 2025

Library of Congress Cataloging-in-Publication Data
Names: Walker, Gavin Robert, author.
Title: Songs of the South African AIDS crisis / Gavin Robert Walker.
Description: New York : Bloomsbury Academic, 2025. | Includes bibliographical references and index.
Identifiers: LCCN 2025013905 (print) | LCCN 2025013906 (ebook) | ISBN 9781666928525 (hardback) | ISBN 9798765154915 (pdf) | ISBN 9781666928532 (epub)
Subjects: LCSH: AIDS (Disease) and the arts—Africa. | AIDS (Disease) and the arts—South Africa. | AIDS (Disease)—Africa—Songs and music. | AIDS (Disease)—South Africa—Songs and music.
Classification: LCC NX180.A36 W35 2025 (print) | LCC NX180.A36 (ebook) | DDC 780/.0362—dc23/eng/20250612
LC record available at https://lccn.loc.gov/2025013905
LC ebook record available at https://lccn.loc.gov/2025013906

ISBN: HB: 978-1-6669-2852-5
ePDF: 979-8-7651-5491-5
eBook: 978-1-6669-2853-2

Typeset by Deanta Global Publishing Services, Chennai, India

For product safety related questions contact productsafety@bloomsbury.com.

To my mother, who taught me to chase dreams.

Contents

Figure

A Note on Style and Terminology

South Africa's history of colonialism, racial segregation, and political disenfranchisement complicates and sensitizes terminology relating to race. During the apartheid years, the population was crudely divided into four racial categories: Black, White, Coloured, and Indian. This terminology continues to be used within official government designations to this day. As a result, this book applies such terms where appropriate in the broader context of the South African AIDS crisis.

Unlike in other parts of the world such as the United States or the United Kingdom, the term "Coloured" does not share the same overwhelmingly negative connotations in South Africa. Introduced as a pseudoscientific catch-all designation for a diversity of peoples (including the indigenous Khoikhoi and San peoples, slaves and political prisoners exiled from Dutch colonies in Southeast Asia, and those of mixed-race heritage), the term has largely been domesticated in contemporary South Africa. While still contested and unresolved, it is widely adopted in reference to the unique cultural identities that have emerged as a result of the country's colonial history.

On a point of style, it has become conventional in recent years to capitalize racial designations across popular, journalistic, and academic print media (although there is some debate on the matter). This book, in accordance with the recommendations of its publisher, follows the guidelines laid out by the *Chicago Manual of Style*, which in a recent online amendment outlined their position in support of the uppercase solution used above.

However, it is understandable that the appearance of the capitalized racial designation "White" may elicit discomfort among some readers as a result of South Africa's long and painful history of White supremacy. This, of course, is not my intention. My decision to capitalize every racial designation (unless reproduced in a quotation) not only follows established convention but seeks to render stylistic decisions such as this powerless to evoke notions of racial superiority. By implementing a consistent uppercase approach, this book treats everyone with equal respect.

Acknowledgments

It may sound like a cliché, but I consider myself something of a dreamer. This simple fact has influenced the course of my life perhaps more than any other. The thing about dreamers is that we follow our instincts in pursuit of our goals with an intensity that often surpasses our current knowledge or abilities. To dreamers, there are no boundaries that cannot be broken nor obstacles that cannot be overcome. But this singular focus comes at a cost; we are susceptible to losing ourselves. The people around us who provide guidance and support are anchors without whom we would lose our way, consumed by our own enthusiasm and hubris. It is for this reason that, to me, this is one of the most important and difficult sections of this book to write. Why? Because it is important to me that I get this right.

This book has been twelve years in the making and is the culmination of countless discussions, interactions, hangouts, interviews, focus groups, observations, and casual chats. Throughout that time, I encountered a great many people to whom I owe my immense gratitude. My appreciation is extended to all those who, through their willingness to accommodate my presence, questions, and wide-eyed ardor, have made this book possible.

In 2012, I stepped through the doors of SOAS, University of London, with a musicological background and little more than a naïve enthusiasm toward beginning my doctoral studies in the anthropology of music. The conceptual material that eventually coalesced into the ideas found in these pages began their journey under the tutelage of noted ethnomusicologist, Professor Angela Impey. It was under her careful mentorship that I was shown the tools to develop and eventually refine the theoretical underpinnings of my work. She provided insightful direction and, where prudent, allowed space for my fledgling ideas to grow. Without her guidance, patience, empathy, and willingness to accommodate my many trips to South Africa, the foundations of this book would not have been possible. She has my greatest respect and admiration as a scholar and a mentor.

My thanks are extended to numerous members (past and present) of the Treatment Action Campaign. Specifically, I owe my gratitude to Mandla Majola, Nkenshani Mavasa, and Fikelephi Dombolo Sithole, who gave their time to share their experiences with me. Additionally, I am indebted to Jack Lewis, whose willingness to assist a complete stranger in connecting with important AIDS advocacy networks demonstrates a warmhearted openness that will remain with me for a long time. Jack put me in contact with Thembeka Majali and Themba Baleni of The Generics, whose experiences and powerful insights were invaluable to understanding the effects of communal singing during the peak of the AIDS epidemic, my deepest gratitude to them both. I must also acknowledge the importance of the work that went into Jack's Community Media Trust AIDS Archive—in collaboration with the University of Cape Town—that documented and meticulously archived much of the Treatment Action Campaign's early activities.

I am grateful to Professor Jan du Toit and the late Professor Jimmie Earl Perry for welcoming my presence at the Africa Centre for HIV/AIDS Management, Stellenbosch University, for much of my time in South Africa. They went above and beyond their roles as affiliate researcher hosts and not only contributed enormously to my project but also to my well-being while spending extended periods of time in what was at the time an unfamiliar country. With the passing of Professor Jimmie Earl Perry in 2018, the AIDS advocacy community of South Africa lost a true titan of compassion, empathy, diplomacy, and talent. He is sorely missed.

My thanks go to the Educational Theatre Company for accepting me into their midst while on tour across the country. I value the memories made during those often exciting and eventful trips. Special mention must be made of Ricardo de Ruiter, Percy Speelman, and Ainé de Vries for accommodating my request to be featured on the cover of this book. My gratitude also goes to Bronwyn Pierce, who graciously drove from Cape Town to Stellenbosch upon my request for an interview in her capacity as the deputy director of the ZAZI campaign and whose perspectives were crucial to unpacking various avenues of audiovisual and mass media AIDS interventions in South Africa.

Portions of this book have reproduced small sections from previously published works—of which I am the sole author—with permission from the publishers. These are "Pulsing Bodies and Embodying Pulse: Musical Effervescence in a South African HIV/AIDS Community Outreach Programme" in the journal *Anthropology & Medicine*, 9 (3), 289–304; "'A Song Is Not Just a Song': Community Mobilisation and Psychosocial Healing in South Africa's AIDS Crisis" in the journal *African Studies*, 80 (3–4), 310–4; and "Music Research in a South African Higher Education Institution" in the journal *Action, Criticism and Theory for Music Education*, 18 (3), 144–71.

My gratitude goes to Professor James Thompson and Dr. Grant Olwage for their invaluable feedback on earlier drafts of this book. Both took time out of their busy schedules to read the entire manuscript; a gesture of generosity that I will not soon forget and hope to repay in the future. I would also like to express my appreciation to Sydney Williams, African Studies editor at Bloomsbury Publishing, for her support for this project from acquisition to publication.

Finally, a book is not simply the work of the author; support is instrumental to success, and I could not have asked for a more encouraging parent than my mother, Nicola Summers. Her unwavering moral, emotional, and practical support throughout my life—especially during the particularly demanding periods of my early academic career—has continuously encouraged me to strive for my ambitions in ways that would be unfathomable in her absence. For this, I will always be grateful.

List of Abbreviations

ACHAM—Africa Centre for HIV/AIDS Management (Stellenbosch University)
AIDS—Acquired Immunodeficiency Syndrome
ALP—AIDS Law Project
ANC—African National Congress
ART—Antiretroviral therapy
ARV—Antiretroviral
AZT—Azidothymidine (an ART)
BEE—Black Economic Empowerment
CMT—Community Media Trust
CWP—Community Work Programme
DMF—Dimethylformamide
EE—Entertainment-education
GEAR—Growth, Employment and Redistribution
HAART—Highly Active Antiretroviral Therapy
HIV—Human immunodeficiency virus
KZN—KwaZulu-Natal (South African Province)
MK—Umkhonto we Sizwe (Spear of the Nation)
MSF—Médecins Sans Frontières/Doctors Without Borders
MTCT—Mother-to-child Transmission
NAPWA—The National Association of People with AIDS
NCGLE—The National Coalition for Gay and Lesbian Equality
NGO—Non-governmental Organization
PAC—Pan African Congress
PLHIV—People Living with HIV
PWA—People with AIDS
RDP—Reconstruction and Development Programme
SANAC—South African National AIDS Council
SAPS—South African Police Service
STI—Sexually Transmitted Infection
TAC—Treatment Action Campaign
TB—Tuberculosis
UN—United Nations
WHO—World Health Organization

1

Antecedent

Stumbling on an uneven and slightly loose cobblestone, sweat is beginning to form across my brow and upper lip. My chest is burning a little from the full sprint I just mustered from the train station to the marketplace—it's not too much further from here. My heart is thumping in my ears and I take a moment to compose myself before continuing on. Walking briskly down the narrow streets that meander around one of central Cape Town's oldest areas, Greenmarket Square, I am acutely aware that I am running late. The train from Stellenbosch, a picturesque university town in the Cape Winelands that I have called home for the past few months, delivered me to the railway station over an hour later than the scheduled arrival time. In hindsight, there were more expedient routes I could have taken.

Having frequented this historic part of the city many times over the past year, the hustle and bustle of the marketplace and the sights and sounds of various street performers floating in and out of my senses is a familiar experience. But there is something decidedly unfamiliar within the usual soundscape today. Barely audible amid the street vendors is another sound, one drifting with indistinct transience upon the hot summer air, distantly struggling for the attention of those within earshot.

The midafternoon sun glints from the windows of nearby cafés where a group of German tourists deliberate over which establishment deserves their vacation custom. I navigate my way through the various souvenir stands arranged in rows from one end of the historic square to the other, offering colorful cell phone cases and South African-themed souvenirs. As I pass by his stall, a young man in dark sunglasses and a red-striped shirt breaks off a conversation with his associates and raises his hand in my direction. Gesturing toward his merchandise, he invites me to browse. I smile but politely decline. The unfamiliar sounds are becoming more distinguished as I cross the square, and I can already hear my final destination, though I cannot see it yet.

The expansive square narrows into a lane, which itself emerges onto a cross-section of asphalt roads, each loomed over by the glass and concrete facades of the city's central business district. Stepping across a busy street at a large set of traffic lights, I turn to find what I am looking for. The increasingly perceptible sounds of vuvuzelas, cheering, and the driving rhythms of hundreds of toyi-toyiing bodies have developed into a full-throated chorus of South African dissent. Upon approach from the direction of the market, and despite the ominous and seemingly intentional visibility of the South African Police Service (SAPS), one might mistake it for a celebration. Such is the nature of much South African performance culture and particularly its music; it can seem joyous and vibrant while simultaneously commanding attention toward dire issues. Four large flagpoles flying the South African national flag mark the grand entrance to the Houses of Parliament, where a large protest is already well underway. Slogans shouted through megaphones—in their characteristically brittle attack—punctuate the energetic scene as a group of ten or more demonstrators toward the front of the rally hold up an enormous black banner, which simply proclaims "PEOPLE OVER PROFITS."

Slightly red-faced and still out of breath, I stand for a moment to take in the scene: an expanse of protesters surrounds the gates of the parliament building, itself presented before the dramatic backdrop of two of the city's most iconic natural landmarks, Lion's Head and Signal Hill. Canorous sounds of anti-apartheid struggle songs sung in four-part harmony resonate off the adjacent buildings and back into the rally, amplifying their vitality. Groups of demonstrators join the call-and-response choruses with their arms thrown toward the sky while others clap and dance jubilantly together to an implied beat.

Whistles and ululations intersperse the melodies as individuals begin to structure themselves into a conga line, further fueling the carnivalesque atmosphere. As more individuals join the dancing line, it becomes a visible manifestation of shared space and time to complement the sonic structuring of bodies. While some scholars have highlighted a tendency toward imbricated and discordant frontiers of sonic niches within the mosaic soundscapes of large-scale demonstrations (Tausig 2019), this protest maintains a level of rhythmic order and collectively directed musicking that eschews such descriptions. It sits in animatedly disobedient contradiction to the rows of unflinching, stony-faced police officers who are scrutinizing the crowd distrustfully. An intimidatingly militarized rampart of washed cornflower blue SAPS uniforms.

Leading the protest is the Treatment Action Campaign (TAC). The AIDS advocacy group has joined with Médecins Sans Frontières (MSF) and other activists to protest the unusually high number of pharmaceutical drug patents accepted every year in South Africa. The country's intellectual property laws allow drug companies to extend their patents through minimal alterations to their medicines' formulas or by combining various drugs into one pill. Such practices, the TAC argues, maintain pharmaceutical company monopolies over expensive medicines while prohibiting the introduction of more affordable generic versions.

I had heard about this protest from a former secretary general of the TAC during a brief chat at Stellenbosch University's Africa Centre for HIV/AIDS Management (ACHAM). The then director of the ACHAM had set up the encounter after one of his many meetings with the AIDS advocacy organization. During much of the time spent conducting the ethnographic research that would eventually manifest as these pages, the ACHAM was not simply an academic center from which I conducted my fieldwork but rather a hub for a network of activists, performing artists, stakeholders, and intellectuals, each determined to make an HIV-free generation a reality.

The locked gates of the Houses of Parliament and considerable police presence seem to represent a physical and metaphorical barrier between South African civil society and those in the elite upper echelons. However, the multiracial protest that fills the courtyard, with the TAC's conspicuous HIV POSITIVE T-shirt—specially made for this event with the slogan "bad patents = death" on the reverse side—as their symbol of unity, is a testament to the progress the country has made from its colonial and apartheid past. It stands in striking contrast to the grandiose gray and black statue of the first prime minister of the Union of South Africa, Louis Botha, directly opposite parliament's gates. Upon its stone perch, declaring Botha as a farmer, warrior, and statesman, it stands with its back facing the parliament, almost as if he cannot bear to watch.

As I mingle among the approximately one thousand-strong crowd—with the struggle song-fueled conga line still dominating the audiovisual landscape of the protest—I sense a growing yet indeterminate state of nebulous and excited animation. My emotions heighten. Pausing for a moment, I am not even sure what emotions I am feeling. Drawn into the sonic environment connecting people with purpose, my pulse quickens as protesters dance around me. The overwhelming urge to move my own body within the flow of the crowd washes over me as lyrical phrases are presented, reformed, and developed, before being enthusiastically and harmoniously returned by the chorus. Each call provides the energy for the response, and each response stimulates the urge to call. Antecedent and consequent sustaining one another in seemingly perpetual sonorous and kinetic motion. I leave the protest with an unusual feeling that I had simultaneously experienced something profoundly animating, yet innocuous and unremarkable.

In the days following the protest, my reflections turn with increasing regularity to questions of how and why songs were able to cultivate such connectivity and emotional energy, a sonic environment in which one might easily lose oneself. While at the same time, the notion that music could exert such a profound influence on people would present itself in my mind as self-evident. I imagine how the scene that I witnessed compares to the early TAC demonstrations at a time when the will of the South African people was pitted against that of the newly formed democratic government. I try to envisage the profound urgency that must have been palpable when those same songs were mobilizing people living with HIV (PLHIV) to make their voices heard at a time when AIDS killed.

Introduction

Songs have been an influential presence throughout the South African HIV/AIDS epidemic. Drawn from a vibrant and diverse cultural history, they have been used to inspire citizens toward AIDS activism and advocacy, facilitate local psychosocial healing, communicate life-saving health information, motivate communities toward healthy behaviors, and promote acceptance of those living with HIV. This book is about those songs and the people who have sung them. It is about how our human propensity for musicality and sonic creativity has been harnessed to realize health, social, legal, and political achievements throughout the epidemic.

While it is common for work such as my own to present a range of harrowing HIV/AIDS statistics during the period in which the research was conducted (from new infections or mother-to-child transmission [MTCT] to deaths from AIDS-related complications), I do not believe that such specificities here will contribute in any meaningful way to what has already been written. What I will state for context, however, is that South Africa emerged in the late 1990s as the epicenter of the global HIV/AIDS pandemic. And, while substantial improvements have been achieved in treatment access and HIV literacy that have resulted in a considerable reduction in preventable deaths, the nation has largely retained that dubious title in the years that have followed.

This book is the result of over a decade of study, analysis, fieldwork, music-making, and human connections. The content of these pages began life as a doctoral thesis that I completed at the School of Oriental and African Studies, University of London. The purpose was to explore the nature and application of song within the context of the AIDS epidemic. While I was not entirely sure exactly what that meant at the time, I was about to begin an ethnographic, empirical, theoretical, and sonorous journey that would culminate in drawing threads of significance between the dizzying variety of creative musical expressions that comprise the historical and ongoing soundscapes of AIDS in South Africa. Based at the ACHAM at Stellenbosch University, I spent much of my time exploring the road less traveled among the anthropological and ethnomusicological scholarship of the AIDS epidemic. While the eastern coastal province of KwaZulu-Natal (KZN) gained notoriety by way of its alarming HIV/AIDS statistics, I spent the majority of my time in the urban townships of the Western Cape—where the number of new HIV infections rivaled those of KZN—as well as in underprivileged rural areas of the Free State and Mpumalanga—all areas where the social, economic, and political determinants of AIDS pose the greatest challenges.

While the scale through which music, and songs in particular, have been adopted for varying purposes in the South African AIDS crisis may be vast, in this book I outline a diverse set of powerful examples of how they have been employed to achieve positive health and social outcomes. The book adopts a perspective that reframes the seemingly disparate applications of song within the crisis as manifestations of the same sets of phenomena operating through the same principles in different contexts and for different purposes. I have termed this phenomenon "musical effervescence."

The approach is derived from French sociologist Émile Durkheim's ([1912] 2008) concept of collective effervescence, a phenomenon in which individuals become physically, affectively, and emotionally animated into quasi-euphoric states through the focused synchronicity of communal interaction rituals. Developing his original theory, this book integrates approaches from the disciplines and subdisciplines of medical anthropology, ethnomusicology, biological anthropology, sociology, and evolutionary musicology to develop a theory of musical effervescence. The phenomenon can be described as a heightened affective state of intersubjectivity facilitated through collective musical experiences. It emerges from the blending of music, purpose, participation, synchronicity, and embodiment. Similar to Durkheim's own observations, hallmarks of musical effervescence include the cultivation of heightened affective states of being and the entrainment of bodies and minds among groups of participants. These affective states may then facilitate the conceptualization of ideal forms of interpersonal and social relationships associated with the particular purpose or goal, and a belief in a world in which those ideals are made manifest, that is to say, a kind of manic creativity among participants of the effervescent assembly.

While Durkheim described song, dance, and rhythmic chant as products of an effervescent assembly, I propose that they can be, and often are, fundamental components in its creation and maintenance. The inherently connective and participatory qualities of music-making within South Africa's unique cultural history unite the applications of song within the AIDS epidemic that are discussed in these pages. Using musical effervescence as a launching point, the book connects such applications within public health interventions, broadly conceived, and provides a framework through which the importance of song to influence social and health outcomes may be better understood.

This theoretical approach emerged as a result of my interactions with HIV/AIDS activists, community choirs, applied theater performers, and mass media campaigns and their audiences. While it may seem at first glance that there are few similarities between instances in which music has been applied within the AIDS crisis that are discussed in this book, the more I experienced and observed, uncanny similarities in behavior—far beyond that of mere coincidence—began to emerge. Singing together in shared purpose seemed to create connections that not only cultivated remarkably similar behavior but also largely transcended profound social, economic, cultural, and ethnic barriers that remain polarizing across South Africa to this day.

While the focus of this book is the application of songs within the South African AIDS crisis, musical effervescence, as a theoretical framework, is not constrained to the conceptual or geographic boundaries of South African songs. Indeed, as the name suggests, it may be applied to many forms of musical activity and across a range of social, linguistic, and cultural contexts. The questions that arise in contemplating the songs that have been—and continue to be—applied within the HIV/AIDS epidemic in South Africa are the same questions that ethnomusicologists, musicologists, philosophers, and theorists have deliberated at various points since antiquity. From the most intimate of private moments to the largest of social movements, musical experiences are often found at the heart of rituals or events that improve our quality of life, social bonds, and well-being. But why? What is it about these experiences that facilitate at the same time both the deeply personal and the fundamentally social? How can music be applicable for such a wide range of outcomes? What can the conception of musical effervescence contribute to our understanding of the arts and social, emotional, or physical wellness? Contemplating potential answers to these questions not only helps to connect the applications of songs within the AIDS crisis through a broad overarching framework of music-driven intersubjectivity but also strengthens the theoretical foundation from which we might understand music beyond the boundaries of this book.

Long-standing musical traditions form a core part of national and cultural identity for many South Africans. From education, initiation rites, coming-of-age rituals, weddings, and sangoma shamanic divinations, the performing arts, and song in particular, are important pillars of social life across the country's many cultures. Considering the importance of song and performance culture in South Africa, it is unsurprising that social expressions and responses to HIV/AIDS involving the arts were common at the height of the epidemic and continue to be to this day. As the country with both the highest population of PHLIV and the largest antiretroviral (ARV) program in the world, AIDS in South Africa has been well-documented across disciplines in the academic literature, which will be discussed later in this chapter.

Despite this abundance of scholarship, however, important phenomena that are fundamental to understanding song and its roles in the epidemic have consistently been overlooked. Some points of contact will help to demonstrate my point. While not the exclusive focus of this book, two of its chapters are dedicated to the TAC. Much has been written about this organization. As the largest AIDS activist and advocacy group in the country, scholars have discussed at length its history and biography, its founding members, their particular brand of activism, and their historic legal challenge that compelled vocal AIDS dissidents in the South African government to make ARV medication available to all. But they have consistently overlooked what I believe to be one of the most powerful tools in their arsenal for social mobilization in the immediate postapartheid era: their use of liberation songs as a rallying cry in the new struggle against HIV/AIDS. These songs were instrumental not only in raising awareness of the burgeoning epidemic at a time when there was no treatment available to South Africans in the public healthcare system but also in raising a nation to its feet to fight, once again, for their basic human rights—the right to life and health.

While the struggle songs that expressed resistance to White minority rule are potent examples, throughout the pages of this book I seek to demonstrate that the power of song as a force for health, political, legal, and social outcomes can be found across a range of creative outputs. Indeed, a further example of song being overlooked can be found within the otherwise abundant literature on the topic of applied theater for health and social change. Applied theater is currently the most popular edutainment approach to presenting information on HIV on the African continent; however, there is a dearth of information relating to the at times crucial roles that songs can, and frequently do, play within the narratives.[1] Despite the wealth of examples of musical responses to crises in South Africa and the irony of being a vocal sonic art, song has been largely silent within the academic literature.

Moreover, much of the anthropological and ethnomusicological explorations of music within the AIDS crisis come in the form of in-depth ethnographies of a particular organization, choir, or other group. Of course, this is a staple format for such research as it provides a sensitive and reflexive method for gaining appropriately situated knowledge. However, while this approach provides tremendously detailed descriptions and analyses of the chosen focus, it also leaves in its wake the unintended consequence of creating islands of expertise within the broader literature. These islands are seldom connected outside of the purview of academic literature reviews. By elucidating the processes through which music may animate us into affectively charged heightened emotional states, musical effervescence provides a theoretical tool through which to draw connections between various forms of music-making. In doing so, this book seeks to address certain gaps in the representation of knowledge and experience within the South African AIDS crisis. It aspires to tell some of the stories that shed light on how song became a consistent presence throughout the varying and disparate expressions, interventions, and responses to the epidemic.

However, while telling such stories and attempting to understand the complexities of the world around us, scholars must be careful of our propensity for oversimplification and categorization. We risk falling into the trap of essentializing peoples and cultures. As scholars of the arts across the African continent have noted, essentialisms from the academy are commonplace (Agawu 2003). As Díaz (2021) has discussed in his recent monograph on the subject, while essentialisms may bestow immutable qualities that bind bodies or phenomena together, they also limit the perception of that which is essentialized to change. It will become clear upon even the most perfunctory reading of this book that a fundamental aspect of the various applications of music within the South African AIDS crisis has been, and continues to be, the creativity and adaptability of both the music and musicians.

Perhaps the most potentially essentializing aspect of this book relates to long-standing associations between African music and collectiveness, expressiveness, spirituality, and social harmony. It is, of course, not my intention to further such tropes. Far from being an exclusively African experience, musical effervescence is a fundamentally human phenomenon (as I will demonstrate in some detail later in Chapter 3). South Africa is the geographic and cultural subject of this book, not because of some outmoded conception of an inherently musical African people but rather due to the country's unique social and political history: one that created the confluence of circumstances that allowed the virus to thrive in a region with a long history of cultural tools with which to combat it.

Injustice and Illness: Connections between the Past and Present

Despite the attempted destruction of a unified Black South African national identity under White minority rule during apartheid, the performing arts were forged into cultural armor and weaponry in the form of struggle songs and other performative expressions of resistance. Generations of oppression have permeated the country's performing arts, with song becoming a powerful catalyst for mobilization and protest. Deployed to comment on and radically reshape the country's social and political landscape throughout the liberation struggle, songs were useful vehicles for opaque coded messages or meanings that could be disseminated relatively quickly among large numbers of people without any significant traceable footprint.

The legacy of struggle and the culture that developed as a result are held in quasi-mythical status in postapartheid South Africa. While this book is not exclusively concerned with the repertoire of struggle songs that has developed over decades, it is important to highlight that it has become largely inseparable from national identity for many South Africans. While apartheid and AIDS seemingly share little outside of their cost in human suffering, until recently, there have been few issues in South Africa's postapartheid history that have highlighted the country's ongoing social, economic, and racial divisions like HIV/AIDS.[2] Not since the fall of White minority rule have South Africa's most vulnerable experienced such a humanitarian catastrophe, and the legacies of apartheid all but ensured the country's grim position as the epicenter of the global AIDS pandemic.

Highly audible and visible discursive linkages include the 46664 AIDS benefit concerts. While this will be explored in significantly more depth in a later chapter, it is still worth mentioning here. Organized by the Nelson Mandela Foundation, this series of concerts adopted its moniker from Nelson Mandela's prison number during his sentence on Robben Island—466/64. By associating one of the most iconic anti-apartheid veterans—himself a symbol in his own right—with the concerts, the former president of South Africa helped to reframe AIDS as the second struggle.

An equally powerful example is that of the juxtaposition of two twelve-year-old boys, separated by a generation, who both needlessly lost their lives at the hands of the South African state apparatus. The first is Hector Pieterson, a schoolboy whose image became synonymous with the brutality of the apartheid regime. Gunned down by the police during the 1976 Soweto uprising, photographer Sam Nzima's now well-recognized shot shows the young boy's limp and bloodstained body being carried away by eighteen-year-old youth activist Mbuyisa Makhubo. Pieterson's distraught sister, Antoinette, is seen following closely behind the two. The second is that of Nkosi Johnson. HIV-positive from birth through MTCT, he rose to prominence in South Africa as a campaigner for HIV/AIDS treatment access until his death from AIDS-related complications in 2001. Visibly ill, he publicly appealed to the South African government to make treatment available as the keynote speaker of the 13th International AIDS Conference. He died shortly after. In the wake of his death, the TAC created banners and posters highlighting the symbolic connections between the two deaths. Symbolic associations between apartheid and AIDS are indicative of an awareness on the part of the South African people of the connections between the suffering of the present and the injustices of the past (Okigbo 2016). Moreover, the creative expressions that have drawn parallels from past atrocities serve as potent reminders of the influence that the creative and performing arts may exert in the face of seemingly insurmountable challenges.

AIDS in Africa: Anthropological and Ethnomusicological Perspectives

A commonly held adage among those who seek to understand the world—regardless of their particular background or approach—is that each of us stands upon the shoulders of giants. This book is not an exception to that rule. Music and health are by no means strangers. The physical and psychological effects of music, typically well-known to musicians, have been documented from as early as 4000 BCE. An oft-cited example is the *Codex Haburami*, or Hallelujah to the Healer, which was sung as payment to Apollo, the chief god of healing in the ancient Greek Olympian pantheon (MacDonald, Kreutz, and Mitchell 2012). The relatively recent developments in medical anthropology and medical ethnomusicology are the latest in a long line of scholarly interest in music (and the arts more generally) and human health and well-being. In writing this book, I have sought to develop the discussions that have their foundations planted firmly within these subdisciplines.

Epidemiological studies and public health reports were the first written accounts of the disease to emerge. Anthropological research on AIDS in South Africa did not peak until the late 2000s and early 2010s, with works such as Didier Fassin's (2007) *When Bodies Remember*, one of the first accounts of the disease that drew explicit connections between apartheid and AIDS. Further notable contributions included approaches to the epidemic that provided a distinctly humanizing approach such as Patricia Henderson's (2011) *A Kinship of Bones*, an ethnographic account of local repertoires of expressing grief and intimacy among PLHIV in the KZN township of Okhahlamba. Mark Hunter's *Love in the Time of AIDS* (2010) presents extended ethnographies of intertwining narratives of love, illness, and economies of intimate relations within rural informal settlements in KZN. Anna Aulette-Root, Floretta Boonzaier, and Judy Aullete's *Women Living with HIV* (2014) focuses on Coloured women's struggle with marginalization, gender inequality, and self-image, drawing from interviews with HIV-positive women in Cape Town. With this flurry of activity came broad acknowledgment of the social, economic, and political determinants and effects of AIDS.

Scholarship in ethnomusicology has been considering music and the performing arts more broadly within healing practices for decades. For example, the work of Steven M. Friedson (1996), whose research explores the local healing and medical practices of the *nchimi* (healers) of the Malawian Tumbuka people, presents a detailed ethnographic account of the lived experiences of healers and their patients. He emphasizes the importance of the human context of Tumbuka healing and the complex intersections between the *nchimi*, music, spirits, and the process of healing. The more formal discipline of medical ethnomusicology developed from similar approaches to music and health and began to gain momentum in the early twenty-first century. The disparate body of research first began to coalesce around the phenomenon of singing for health and well-being that examined music as a therapeutic and social expression of health/illness (see MacDonald, Kreutz, and Mitchell 2013; Barz 2006; Koen, Barz, and Brummel-Smith 2008; McNeill 2011; Kauffmann and Lindauer 2004; McConnell 2020; Walker 2018; Barz and Cohen 2011). Indeed, while traditionally practiced in clinical settings, music therapy has also recently broadened the horizons of its focus in an emerging subfield of community music therapy (Pavlicevic and Ansdell 2004; Stige and Aarø 2011; Stige, Ansdell, Elefant and Pavlicevic 2010; Ansdell, DeNora and Wilson 2016). Further, recent clinical studies have begun to explore music and music-making within patient-focused health interventions, specifically around mental health and dementia (Clare and Camic 2019; Harrison et al. 2010). But while the interest in music and its relationship with human health and well-being is increasing, scholarship on musicking experiences in the context of public health promotion remains underdeveloped (Lemieux, Fisher, and Pratto 2008; Yoshida et al. 2013; Stewart and Irons 2018).

There are a number of medical ethnomusicology texts that are worth noting for their contribution to the foundation of this book. These have generally followed the broad approach of the medical humanities (or health humanities as it is sometimes referred to) to help bridge what can, at times, be a sizeble gap between biomedicine and diagnoses on the one hand, and the people whose lives are affected by illness on the other (Bleakley 2013, 2015). Koen's (2009) position that healing or transformation (physical or spiritual) is intimately interwoven within personal sensitivities, values, norms, consciousness, and "engaged and propagated through one's body and being," forms an important pillar on which recent AIDS-related medical ethnomusicology discourses rest (156). Rather than focusing predominantly on overall health trends or biomedical solutions, although of course these are discussed, these works have shifted the focus toward, but not limited to, coping with HIV and loss through songs and community music-making (Alviso 2011; Eller-Isaacs 2011; Cole 2011), living with stigma and violence (Aulette-Root, Boonzaier, and Aulette 2014), and public health education and social change through music and the performing arts (Bourgault 2003; Barz 2006; van Buren 2011; Reed 2011; McNeill 2011).

Perhaps one of the earliest and most significant of such ethnographies was conducted in Uganda by ethnomusicologist Gregory Barz. His book *Singing for Life* (2006) explores methods employed by rural Ugandan communities to educate, communicate, and cope with HIV/AIDS, what he states as "the role of music in efforts to shout in Uganda" (215). The "shout" became a slogan and device created to aggressively break a culture of silence that emerged around the disease all over the continent. The concept of using music to break prevailing cultures of silence on the subject of AIDS has been applied to the South African epidemic and will become important later in this book.

There were a number of reasons why Barz's work stood out both from the ethnomusicological scholarship of the time and research on HIV/AIDS in Africa. Barz made strong connections between local knowledge and the ritual systems in place for disseminating that knowledge, and the biomedical information involved in effective HIV prevention. This is something that McNeill (2011) would go on to note was still being largely ignored in South Africa several years later. Barz highlighted the potential benefits of integrating such biomedical information into the preexisting local structures of knowledge. These localized approaches to health and healing, often through music, drumming, dance, and theater performances, were positioned as complementary to biomedical information in rural communities with little access to medicine or other health resources.

Singing for Life navigates a number of narratives and dialogues that include first-person reflections of coping with HIV and interviews with individuals—mostly women—who utilize various culturally specific social advocacy techniques in order to transfer knowledge, promote health education, and empower those already living with HIV. Barz, like many others, points out that during the height of the epidemic, a significant number of women in both Uganda (and indeed South Africa) were unable to practice the safe sex health advice so often presented by government and NGO HIV prevention initiatives due to their subordinate status within sexual and marital relationships (Barz 2006; McNeill 2011; Hunter 2010). Thus, appropriation of performance art provided a culturally appropriate vehicle for such advice to be disseminated.

Barz's (2006) work also began to open up discussions around the potential therapeutic properties of music performance outside of the clinical settings of music therapy within the context of AIDS in Africa. In one such example, he writes of sitting in on one group of women who danced ceremonial courtship dances to drummed rhythms, as one of the women, Mama Noelina, describes: "Look at them. It makes them feel better when they dance. They're *dancing their disease*!" (78, emphasis already present). This focus on community-based therapy through performance has gone on to become a prominent theme in not only my own work (Walker 2021a) but also other scholars such as Austin Okigbo, whose book *Music, Culture and the Politics of Health* (2016) explored the formation and culture surrounding the now-famous Siphithemba HIV-positive choir in South Africa.

Focusing specifically on South Africa, another significant contribution to the literature on HIV/AIDS and music in Africa comes from Fraser McNeill's *AIDS, Politics, and Music in South Africa* (2011). While most previous scholarship on South African music had focused on the country's rich musical heritage, exploring the many divergent histories that have come to characterize its sounds, including segregation and disempowerment prior to and during apartheid, labor migration, and songs in political struggle (Coplan 1985; Ballantine 1993; Erlmann 1991, 1999), McNeil's work was one of the first to draw connections between the country's performance culture and the epidemic.

McNeill focuses largely on the impact of the epidemic on socio-sexual relationships in postapartheid rural South Africa, dealing with peer education and the manner in which knowledge is presented, represented, and disseminated in the old Venda homeland in what is now the Limpopo Province of South Africa. In a similar vein to *Singing for Life*, McNeill (2011) explores various local methods that are used to pass on knowledge, notably young girls' initiations into womanhood. He argues that, in Venda, knowledge is associated with experience and as a result, information is passed down from the elder to the younger generation. The conception of experience as knowledge, however, creates problems in dealing with negative or stigmatized life issues such as sex, death, or disease. In such cases, rituals, including song and dance, may create a safe space in which such knowledge may be given and received. As a result of these views, he states that knowledge can be dangerous in Venda, arguing that "potentially hazardous information, such as that pertaining to sexual health or death, is conventionally transferred through lyrics of songs in highly prescribed ritual contexts, under the protection of ancestral hierarchy or a Christian God" (154). Music, in this case, creates a degree of separation from the subject matter. This underscores the need to understand local conceptions of knowledge and the potentially damaging effects of disrupting them. Thus, in such situations, improperly formulated external information runs the risk of being harmful.

McNeill notes that the peer educators, who are often young women—those affected most significantly by HIV/AIDS in Venda and South Africa in general—are largely shunned by the community by virtue of their biomedical knowledge, which the community leaders do not possess and which is being disseminated outside of the safe environment of the initiations. Indeed, similar issues are noted by anthropologist Susan Levine (2007) when she suggests that popular expressions of disbelief toward HIV/AIDS-related information are used by many in South Africa, Lesotho, and Mozambique to distance themselves from the disease, and the moral judgment and stigma associated with it. In an attempt to circumvent hierarchical systems of knowledge transfer, the Venda peer educators employ music as a method of engaging people. By employing well-known and locally resonant songs, they invoke religious, political, and social sentiment and allegiances as buffers to soften the introduction of dangerous knowledge of HIV/AIDS and condom use. McNeill explains that by adopting such genres, the biomedical information is cloaked in "Vendaness." Thus, culturally resonant music may help to legitimize the introduction of new knowledge within contexts that are usually hostile toward information not recognized within local frameworks.

McNeill's research presents an account of a rural South African approach to the epidemic and usefully illustrates a number of ways in which music and dance are applied within competing narratives of health and illness. *AIDS, Politics and Music in South Africa* is one of the few in-depth ethnographies of South African AIDS prevention that illustrates the difficulties in introducing unmediated information into local systems of understanding health and illness.

By approaching the subject of HIV/AIDS by way of detailed and long-term ethnographies, these studies present a thoroughly human experience of the health crisis in Africa. These ethnomusicological accounts largely remove themselves from medical accounts that favor statistical analyses and numerical surveys, or similar forms of quantitative data gathering (Maher 2002; Fordham 2015), for more personal and reflexive encounters with their interlocutors. For anthropologists and ethnomusicologists, this focus on people and experience over numbers is nothing new, but it has equally served to refresh discourses on the African AIDS crisis, which was largely saturated with biomedical accounts, while generally overlooking the epidemic's marked economic, political, and historical determinants and personal stories.

An approach that many of the aforementioned works share in common is their framing of music and the performing arts as a culturally appropriate vehicle through which to introduce health information. This book builds upon this foundation and is situated within the nexus of overlapping accounts of, and approaches to, the South African AIDS epidemic by documenting and analyzing a multitude of applications of music within the crisis. It positions music as an important methodological device within HIV/AIDS interventions (broadly conceived) and musical effervescence as an analytical tool that may be employed to understand the mechanics of collective music-making for health and social outcomes.

The ethnographic vignette that opens this chapter, and indeed the book as a whole, serves two distinct purposes. The first is to illustrate the highly animating, connective, emotive, and energizing properties of songs and singing among groups of people that encapsulate the overarching theoretical narrative of this book. The TAC, as will be discussed in Chapters 6 and 7, harnessed these properties to great effect to propel their movement for access to HIV medication in the late 1990s and early 2000s. The second purpose is to introduce the ethnographic style that will be employed throughout the majority of this book. In doing so, I join the ranks of anthropologists and ethnomusicologists who have firmly situated their work within the messiness of lived experience.

Themes and Chapters

There are three main themes that this book addresses. The first is HIV awareness and prevention. It explores efforts to break the silence of HIV/AIDS as well as the history of celebrity advocacy and the mega-events of the 1980s (Band Aid, Live Aid, etc.) as precursors for the kinds of performance-based and audiovisual HIV awareness media that have become common in South Africa. The theme positions the 46664 AIDS benefit concerts of the early 2000s and the celebrity-endorsed music videos that emerged to promote HIV/AIDS awareness as South Africa's answers to Live Aid and Band Aid, and discusses the employment of these methods—and their perceived impact—within the crisis. The theme also examines the role of songs and musical effervescence with applied theater and discusses the significant influence that music can have on the success or failure of such interventions. The second theme considers the role of song within social mobilization, activism, and advocacy. This theme focuses specifically on the

TAC and their use of tactical social marketing, rights-based activism, liberation culture, and struggle songs. The theme explores the use of reappropriated liberation songs to galvanize musical effervescence among large numbers of activists during rallies and protests not only to draw people to their cause but also to maintain the momentum of the movement through entrainment in rhythm, pulse, and communal music-making. Song is cultural armor among South Africa's struggle veterans, and the tools of liberation are a formidable force for activism, advocacy, healing, and social change. The book draws connections between two of South Africa's most enduring tragedies, apartheid and AIDS. It outlines how the meticulously implemented racial oppression and barbaric human rights abuses created a perfect storm in which HIV could flourish among the country's disenfranchised masses. But the same cultural weaponry that was deployed to overthrow White minority rule was reappropriated and refocused against the legacies of oppression. The final theme involves songs as community-based therapy. The theme explores communal singing as a form of therapeutic space through which participants can connect with one another spatially and temporally to encourage the healing of the psychological, social, and emotional burdens of AIDS. To do this, the theme focuses on The Generics, an HIV-positive choir associated with the TAC.

Chapter 2 presents some of the key details relating to the history and political economy of AIDS in South Africa. It outlines the symptoms of structural violence as legacies of White minority rule and racial segregation. These symptoms, in turn, are reframed as determinants of HIV transmission among some of the country's most economically vulnerable populations. In doing so, the chapter draws direct links between apartheid and AIDS. The chapter provides the contextual information relevant to the discussions relating to the abundance of health communication strategies that were implemented by civil society organizations in response to state-sponsored misinformation, the emergence of the TAC as a vocal counterweight to state-sponsored AIDS denialism, and the application of communal singing for hope and psychosocial healing as a response to the lack of government support for antiretroviral therapy (ART) in the national health system.

Based on French sociologist Émile Durkheim's ([1912] 2008) concept of collective effervescence—a collective emotional state of synchronized intersubjectivity—Chapter 3 outlines the conceptual framework through which the book will approach the use of songs throughout the AIDS epidemic. By drawing together phenomenological, sociological, psychological, paleo-musicological, ethnomusicological, and anthropological theories and applying them to communal music-making, the chapter presents a distinct approach to understanding the psychological and physiological influence of collective musical experiences. The chapter argues that highly animated and emotionally charged states of being may be cultivated through communal singing or participation in musical activities, and that such responses to collective music-making emerge from some of the most fundamental of biopsychosocial processes that have developed throughout human evolution.

Chapter 4 continues to frame the discussions of the book by providing contextual information relating to the cultural importance of music in traditional education, initiation rites, weddings, and sangoma shamanic divinations in South Africa. It discusses the use of songs within the liberation struggle and the weaponization of local performance culture to resist White minority rule throughout the colonial and apartheid eras. The chapter provides a foundation for later discussions that explore the reappropriation of the culturally resonant and emotionally powerful repertoire of songs for the purposes of mobilizing local communities toward AIDS activism and their use as a therapeutic aid for psychosocial healing and community support.

In Chapter 5, I provide an overview of the HIV/AIDS-related informative entertainment initiatives employed both within communities and throughout the South African media landscape. The chapter discusses edutainment TV dramas, celebrity advocacy, and applied theater and explores the influence of Live Aid and other celebrity advocacy initiatives on the messaging applied to the South African AIDS crisis. It positions the 46664 AIDS benefit concerts of the early 2000s and the music videos that are discussed later in Chapter 9 as legacies of the humanitarian mega concerts and music videos of the 1980s, deploying similar mega-event and star power approaches as Live Aid and Band Aid. In doing so, I argue that by failing to draw sufficient connections between the musicking experience and the purpose of the performances, the concerts were largely unable to cultivate musical effervescence, resulting in poor translation of messaging to outcomes. It also provides the contextual information required for discussions relating to mass media and applied theater health interventions found in subsequent chapters.

Focusing specifically on their adoption of singing, struggle culture, and performance-based activism, Chapter 6 explores the activities of South Africa's largest AIDS advocacy and activist organization, the TAC. The chapter discusses various mismanaged state responses to the AIDS crisis under the Mandela and Mbeki presidencies and the resultant mistrust that developed between civil society and the government. It then explores the tactical social marketing approaches that the TAC used to gain support across racial and ethnic lines by enveloping their own struggle for health justice in the culture and music of the struggle against apartheid. It draws upon ethnographic data collected from contemporary protests, interviews with founding TAC members, and archival material from the University of Cape Town's Community Media Trust (CMT) AIDS Archive to argue that the TAC's activism deployed musical effervescence to invigorate the struggle for access to ARV medication.

Chapter 7 explores the ways in which collective singing in choirs has provided community-level support and psychosocial healing for those affected and infected by HIV during a period of South African history in which life-saving ARV medications were not available. The chapter discusses The Generics, the HIV-positive choir associated with the TAC. The chapter presents the story of the choir as well as accounts from former choir members regarding the role of The Generics in community therapy. It frames the connective synchronicity, and the physiological and emotional responses, as manifestations of musical effervescence insofar as the communal singing aided the choir members in conceptualizing an ideal form of reality, one in which medication is available to all South Africans and their health and lives are preserved. The chapter analyzes a number of the songs that were reappropriated from South Africa's liberation struggle.

In Chapter 8, I build upon the discussion of edutainment in Chapter 5 to explore the role of songs with applied theater for HIV/AIDS awareness and prevention. Drawing from the case study *Lucky, the Hero!*—a mini-musical organized by Stellenbosch University's Africa Centre for HIV/AIDS Management—the chapter ethnographically explores the deployment of musical effervescence within applied theater for HIV/AIDS awareness, prevention, and testing in several rural communities across South Africa. The chapter highlights the importance of the embodiment of sound within musical effervescence and the fragility with which those experiences are made and unmade.

Chapter 9 develops the themes introduced in the opening chapters by discussing edutainment and mass media HIV/AIDS initiatives. Specifically, it analyzes the content of a high-profile HIV/AIDS-related music video to examine the mechanisms utilized to raise awareness around HIV transmission, alter behaviors, and cultivate social change. The chapter discusses the *ZAZI* music video, an HIV/AIDS and gender-based violence campaign released in 2013 by the South African National AIDS Council (SANAC) and Johns Hopkins University. The analysis is then bolstered by questionnaires and focus groups with young South Africans to explore the reception of the music video. The chapter introduces the term "transient pseudo-effervescence" to explain a phenomenon of heightened motivation for action and belief in ideals that may be reached while exposed to audiovisual media. Transient pseudo-effervescence helps to explain why the models utilized by Band Aid have been so successful within the limited scope of raising funds for humanitarian purposes.

The final chapter draws together the various discussions threaded throughout these pages. The purpose of the book is to not only highlight the multitude of musical responses to the South African HIV/AIDS epidemic but also to propose a new approach through which to explore the use of song within the crisis. The seemingly disparate applications of songs discussed in this book share important ingredients for their success (which in this context is determined by the health and social outcomes that they have helped to facilitate). It is their participatory and culturally resonant nature that so deeply influences those who experience them. These, I argue, are fundamental to the phenomenon that unites these applications of song, musical effervescence. While musical effervescence is not a uniquely African phenomenon, the power of song in South Africa is rooted in local ways of being that predate European colonial conquest, the subsequent domestication of colonial influences, and a proud tradition of resistance and cultural armament. Song has been deployed for generations to influence the collective South African political economy. Far more than a simple soundtrack to life, song in South Africa has been a tonic through which to heal and a weapon through which to overthrow tyranny. Wielded through generations by sangoma, local leaders, freedom fighters, and community activists, these songs are saturated with the lived experiences of those for whom freedom was everything. Those same cries for freedom and justice continue to echo through the familiar melodies, regardless of who is singing or what they are singing about. The chapter draws together the various threads of this book to demonstrate the socio-musical mechanics of musical effervescence as it has manifested within the various struggles for life, love, social acceptance, information, and healing in South Africa's AIDS crisis.

Notes

1 Some headway is being made on this front with emerging scholarship proposing the application of a broadly conceived folk media, in which performances are framed within the vernaculars of local community performance culture, including music (Chinyowa 2009). My own work has called for increased interdisciplinarity between music studies and applied theater (Walker 2024).

2 South Africa's acute social and economic injustices, as well as the failure to adequately transform the country's apartheid-era structural inequities that continue to marginalize large swathes of its population, have been highlighted by sweeping student protests and calls for decolonization that emerged in the mid-2010s (Walker 2019; Jansen 2017).

2

The Poisoning of the Poor

A Historical Political Economy of AIDS in South Africa

The story of South Africa's HIV/AIDS epidemic stands as unique within sub-Saharan Africa, and the history of the region plays an important role in understanding the magnitude of the crisis. The legacies of imperialism, settler colonialism, and the system of racially motivated social engineering known as apartheid have continued to exert influence over the lives and health of South Africans into the present day. The first manifestations of the AIDS crisis largely coincided with the collapse of this system and the first truly democratic dispensation of the mid-1990s. This unfortunate timing would significantly influence the trajectory of events that would ultimately culminate in South Africa emerging as the epicenter of the global AIDS pandemic.

The title of this chapter highlights a potent representation of fear and mistrust wrought from hundreds of years of oppression, political disenfranchisement, and violence. The Poisoning of the Poor refers to a commonly held belief early in the epidemic that a jealous and resentful White minority were attempting to poison the country's Black majority after losing control of the state (Henderson 2011). While poison may not be at the heart of the health crisis, the structural inequalities that put the nation's most economically disadvantaged communities at higher risk of HIV infection are considerably more dangerous in their scope and risk to public health. Engaging with the events that led South Africa to become vulnerable to HIV/AIDS, the histories of subjugation, and the various political and economic determinants of the epidemic demonstrates the issues that have led to the "poisoning" of South Africa's poor (Walker 2021a).

The legacies of colonialism and apartheid still loom large. Persistent social and economic inequality continue to be some of the primary determinants of HIV infection. The contemporary manifestations of past injustices mandate that any analysis of the AIDS epidemic be historically situated within the context of decisions made by the powerful and how they have come to affect the powerless (Farmer 2005). In addition, there is a moral dimension to scholarship that engages with such ordeals. HIV has devastated families and individuals in South Africa. As a scholar, ethnographer, and human being, it is important to me—and many others before me who have done similar work—that such suffering is not only acknowledged but also accurately represented and contextualized within the overarching economic, political, and social environment that culminated in such a catastrophe (Decoteau 2008; Farmer 1992; Biehl 2005).

The discussions in this chapter are broad and cross a range of different, yet very much interrelated topics. While an exhaustive account is beyond the scope of these pages, each must be addressed in order to properly contextualize the ongoing HIV/AIDS epidemic. Connecting the causal links between large-scale sociopolitical forces (poverty, racism, violence, structural inequality, etc.) and individual distress, suffering, and disease highlights the interconnectedness of history, political economy, and lived experiences of AIDS in South Africa, insofar as such outcomes are the embodiment of these forces (Farmer 1999, 2005, 2009; Posel 2008; Hunter 2010). In short, when it comes to HIV/AIDS in South Africa, history matters, and to tell this story, we have to go back rather a long time.

Migration and Economic Exploitation During the Colonial and Apartheid Eras

In 1795, the British took control of the Cape of Good Hope from the Dutch state. The early nineteenth century saw the British extend control over the region with the expansion of the Cape and Natal Colonies. This resulted in a number of frontier wars, including conflicts with the indigenous Xhosa and Zulu peoples, as well as earlier Dutch settlers (or Afrikaners) (Ross 1999). The discovery of gold and diamonds in the interior of what was then Afrikaner-administered land motivated the British to occupy these areas and begin extracting their mineral wealth (Thompson 2001). The discovery intensified preexisting, but still largely informal, racial segregation exercised by earlier settlers as cheap Black labor was used to mine the deposits. Trains from as far north as Uganda brought thousands of laborers to what is now the wider Johannesburg and Witwatersrand areas, creating a migrant labor system that is still, in many ways, operating today, though on a much smaller scale (Jeeves 1985; Segatti 2011).

By 1910, the first recognizable borders of the contemporary South African state had been drawn through the British annexation of the Zulu kingdom and the two Afrikaner republics (Transvaal and Orange Free State) (Ross 1999). The Union of South Africa, a dominion of the British Empire, was governed by a coalition parliament consisting of the Afrikaners and the British. The first legislative blow to those not of European descent passed by this parliament came in the form of the Native Land Act (1913). Although this was not the first law to limit the rights of indigenous groups in the previous colonies or republics, it was the first law to formally strip people of the right to be self-sufficient (Kallen 2011). The Act was designed to regulate Black ownership of arable land in the newly formed country and further prevented them from renting farms from European farmers (Feinstein 2005; Higginson 2014). The result of such legislation, and the introduction of taxation, was that Black South Africans had little choice other than to find work outside of lands they had previously depended on. Such work was found in few places other than the gold and diamond mines. Indigenous communities were allocated small plots of predominantly nonarable land, large enough to "justify" extremely low wages, while small enough to guarantee they could not be entirely self-sufficient, thus ensuring a constant flow of labor to the mines. As one historian suggests, "the final outcome of the whole process was that, for the African people of South Africa, land was no longer abundant; in areas they could still own, land was scarce and it was labor that was plentiful" (Feinstein 2005, 48).

The South African government and industry interests engineered the migrant labor system to structure and stratify society (Lurie 2010). It effectively served to break down the social fabric of rural South African life, with the family at its core (Hunter 2010), by destabilizing rural family structures. The system largely prevented Black men from settling in urban areas while simultaneously forcing them into long periods of time working away from their families, often housed in enormous single-sex accommodation. Due to sets of pernicious influx control laws, the separation of parents and children was particularly common in rural areas, where both men and women inevitably sought work beyond their home areas. South Africa's children and youth have thus long been involved in fluid childcare arrangements whereby not only adults but also children have been mobile in pursuit of schooling, work, health care, and political safety (Henderson 2011).

Population displacement, migrant labor, and geographic mobility have been identified across the developing world as risk factors for the transmission of infections such as HIV and tuberculosis (TB) (Lurie 2010). Indeed, European colonialism in Africa in the nineteenth century, and the labor systems designed and implemented by those administrations, paved the way for what some researchers have described as a "perfected storm" for the sub-Saharan African HIV/AIDS epidemic (Faria et al. 2014). Rapid European colonial expansion and industrialization across the African continent created conditions of interconnectedness—through vast rail networks—and economic exploitation that have allowed the virus to flourish. As with all colonial exploits, the interests of the governing European state and private commerce took precedence over indigenous populations, and thus subjugated peoples saw very little of the capital flowing to, and materials flowing from the region, causing enormous social imbalances along racial lines (Hunter 2002).

The mineral wealth-based economy of South Africa's mines created the need for an almost exclusively male workforce. Since the mines were often far from laborers' home communities, with contracts often lasting for several months, coupled with new disposable incomes and few economic opportunities for women, it is unsurprising that a booming sex trade flourished in and around mining areas (Hongoro, Tadele, and Kloos 2013). A combination of the presence of ulcerative diseases—such as syphilis from sex work—and poor hygiene practices in sexual health clinics appears to have contributed to the rapid expansion of HIV across the sub-Saharan continent (Pépin 2021). In terms of South Africa's current HIV/AIDS crisis, movement and intimate person-to-person contact are at the forefront of any capacity for the virus to spread, and the migrant labor system that was streamlined by consecutive racist governments contributed significantly to the epidemic.

During the 1948 general election, the National Party took control of the Union of South Africa and immediately began to enshrine the dominant position of White South Africans into law through what it referred to as apartheid (translated from Afrikaans to mean "separateness"). When considering the structures that directly and indirectly influence South Africa's current HIV/AIDS epidemic, it is difficult to overstate the ongoing legacy of apartheid. This legislated system of segregation and racially motivated social engineering cultivated conditions that made Black and Coloured South Africans far more likely to be living in poverty and without marketable skills or access to education than their White counterparts (Home 2005).

Throughout the latter half of the twentieth century, South Africa's apartheid regime increasingly restricted the civil liberties of Black South Africans through the enforcement of racially discriminatory laws. The Population Registration Act (1950), which introduced identity cards that stated an individual's race, enshrined racial classifications in law and restricted the movement of all those not of European descent. Further legislation went on to prohibit different racial groups from living within the same "location" (Group Areas Act 1950), romantic or sexual relationships between different races (Immorality Act 1950), and interracial marriage (Prohibition of Mixed Marriages Act 1949), as well as segregate public and private amenities (Reservation of Separate Amenities Act 1953) and education (Bantu Education Act 1953).

The laws passed by the apartheid regime continued and intensified existing exploitative labor conditions, and by the 1970s, the government had begun to move Black South Africans to what it termed "Bantustans" or "homelands" (Beck 2000). These were rural areas mostly devoid of natural resources into which large swathes of the country's ethnic groups were forced to live, thus dividing the Black majority of South Africa's population along ethnic lines, stripping them of citizenship, and creating conditions in which economic success was nearly impossible (Kivnick 1990). Further forced removals were carried out within major metropolitan areas, uprooting families and livelihoods often with little to no warning. The result of such action was the creation of townships and large underprivileged informal settlements on the outskirts of urban centers, as Black South Africans settled as close as legally allowed to the cities in order to find work (Hunter 2007).

Resistance to minority rule was organized by a number of different organizations and took many forms, from peaceful protests to civil disobedience. To simplify, in response to increasing restrictions on civil liberties and racist policies, a collective movement, headed by the African National Congress (ANC) and labor unions, increasingly challenged the apartheid state. By the 1960s, the exiled paramilitary wing of the ANC, *Umkhonto we Sizwe* (MK), began attacking critical civilian infrastructure. In the decades that followed, the ANC continued to step up its organization and encouragement of civil disobedience campaigns and industry strikes in an effort to make the state ungovernable. These efforts resulted in a state of emergency being declared in 1985. By 1990, then-president F. W. de Klerk was impelled to negotiate an end to apartheid. This saw the unbanning of the ANC, the release of Nelson Mandela from prison, and multiracial and fully democratic elections by 1994. White minority rule had officially ended.

Poverty and the Economy of Intimacy: Inequality and Neoliberalism in Postapartheid South Africa

For many, South Africa's transition to democracy, avoidance of civil war, and the ANC's exemplary rhetoric of reconciliation and transformation after decades of legislated institutional racism were a triumph (Fassin 2007; Robins 2008). However, the ills of the past—and indeed their continued impact on the present—cannot simply be relegated to the confines of official institutions such as the Truth and Reconciliation Commission or Apartheid Museum, if they are to be overcome (Fassin 2007). Indeed, the haste to celebrate South Africa's liberation risks overlooking the lack of social and economic mobility the country has experienced since. Anthropologist Steven Robins (2005) refers to this as the fetishizing of first-generation human rights, such as freedoms from discrimination, at the expense of second-generation socioeconomic rights. Indeed, the country's AIDS crisis reveals that while great strides were made in the 1990s to achieve civil liberties, this did not translate into social equality, and though political violence ceased, structural violence did not (Fassin 2007).

It would be an oversimplification, however, to suggest that South Africa has not made advances toward a more economically equitable society. Prior to 1994, the clear definition between the "haves" and "have nots" was drawn distinctly along racial lines, whereas, in postapartheid South Africa, these lines have begun to blur (Bottomley 2012). An emerging Black elite and low-income White communities allude to the gradual weakening of social and economic structures of privilege that were once indistinguishable from race. Further, as I have already mentioned in Chapter 1, I spent much of my time in South Africa based at the ACHAM at Stellenbosch University, formerly a predominantly Afrikaans-speaking institution, historically restricted only to those of European descent. For over two decades, the center has been actively involved in combating a national health crisis that disproportionately affects the lives of Black and Coloured South Africans. However, despite some moderate advancement in fiscal empowerment and social welfare, South Africa remains economically polarized (van der Berg 2006).

As a theoretical tool, structural violence provides a framework through which to examine the social machinery of oppression (Farmer 2004). It describes conditions in which members of a certain social order are subjected to various forms of systematic humiliation, acts of violence, oppression, or suffering. Socioeconomic inequality is one of the most substantial propellants of HIV/AIDS in South Africa. It bears consequence throughout a variety of determinants, including education, migration, and substance abuse (Walker 2022a). Poverty and AIDS are intimately linked as types of structural violence inflicted upon South Africa's most vulnerable through historical and ongoing oppression (Henderson 2011).

Perhaps the most visible manifestations of this are the informal settlements noted earlier in this chapter that frequently can be found on the periphery of major metropolitan centers. The settlements comprise large areas of makeshift housing, usually without access to basic sanitation or amenities, in which much of the nation's urban poor reside. Medical anthropologist João Biehl (2005) refers to these areas as "zones of abandonment" (4), insofar as it is in such places that the voiceless and marginalized reside, largely ignored by the state and on the fringes of society. While zones of abandonment may be identified in a number of economically unequal societies and often develop organically in response to a variety of structural factors, South Africa's informal settlements hold the dubious distinction of being intentionally architected. Many of these zones of abandonment were areas either in which populations of Black or Coloured South Africans settled to be closer to the cities at a time when they were not permitted to live in them or areas in which they were forcibly placed.

South Africa's zones of abandonment highlight tremendous economic disparities that are still largely drawn along racial lines. In the years following the end of the apartheid system, optimism for the country's social and economic development ran high, characterized by the rhetoric of the rainbow nation that was no longer isolated from the global community. However, this development was slow to materialize. Instead, the ANC's economic policies in the immediate postapartheid era reflected a shift toward a more neoliberal economic model, one that favored privatization of public services, free-market capitalism, and reductions in public spending.

This neoliberal direction is particularly visible within South Africa's healthcare system. In the aftermath of the country's liberation, the ANC released their 1994 National Health Plan, part of the Reconstruction and Development Programme (RDP), that outlined a state-run, democratic, and equitable national health service. However, it soon became apparent that such laudable goals would be impeded by fiscal policy and budget constraints. By 1996, the Growth, Employment and Redistribution (GEAR) strategy, which implemented fiscal restraint, privatization of industries and services, and export-oriented production, was already substantially obstructing the kind of redistribution outlined in its predecessor, the RDP, and distancing itself from previous goals of social welfare (Robins 2005; Baker 2010; Narsiah 2002). One of the major issues with South Africa's neoliberal fiscal policy direction was that free markets are motivated by sets of concerns far removed from equity, access, and service to the general public.

South Africa's record following its transition to full democracy is at times strikingly at odds with the ANC's original raison d'être and the principles outlined in the Freedom Charter, a statement of intent adopted in 1955 by the South African Congress Alliance, a collection of civil rights groups comprising the ANC and its allies. The Freedom Charter can easily be interpreted through a lens of national redistribution of the country's resources and the cultivation of a more equitable society, a document that outlines the foundations of a South Africa in which the state looms large (Satgar 2012). Indeed, South Africa's postapartheid constitution was largely hailed at the time of its certification as one of the most progressive in the world.

The reality for many South Africans in the years following the end of apartheid, however, was often quite far removed from the one envisioned both in the Freedom Charter and the country's liberal constitution (von Lieres 2005; Robins 2008). The economic and labor policies of the postapartheid state have, at times, been so at odds with its claim to developmental status that some scholars have dismissed such rhetoric as "propagandistic and declaratory" (Satgar 2012, 37). The former militant language of revolution, socialism, and national liberation was replaced with less threatening keywords such as transformation, citizenship, empowerment, and nation-building. In short, upon taking control of Pretoria, the ANC was "rudely reminded of the limits of political power in a country characterized by centuries of social and economic inequality and racial domination" (Robins 2008, 3). Postliberation South Africa's mixed economy sits on a fault line between its implicit commitment to social welfare (as a result of its roots as a liberation movement) on the one hand and free-market economic policies on the other, what von Lieres (2005) refers to as "an explosive mixture of liberal and non-liberal politics" (22).

The surge of HIV infections in the years following the end of White minority rule represents a failure of successive governments to redress the political and economic injustices of apartheid and colonialism (Decoteau 2008). South Africa remains to this day one of the most economically unequal countries in the world. Enormous discrepancies in wealth lead to an uneven distribution of infection and access to medical treatment (Hunter 2007). Without the kinds of economic restructuring that could have prevented the spread of infectious diseases such as HIV/AIDS or TB, South Africa's poor communities were placed on the front lines of a burgeoning epidemic.

Symptoms of Structural Violence: Sexual Violence, Alcoholism, and Transactional Relationships

South Africa has one of the highest rates of sexual violence in the world. Estimates suggest that the incidence of rape at the height of the AIDS crisis in 1999—when South Africa was experiencing the peak of its new HIV infections—was as high as 1.6 million (du Toit 2014). As the primary mode of HIV transmission is through sexual contact, the high incidence of rape further strengthened the epidemic's grip on the country, with victims of sexual violence at risk of infection.

HIV prevalence has been found to be significantly higher within the country's zones of abandonment, strongly indicating a causal relationship between poverty, historical trauma, and risk of HIV transmission (Shisana et al. 2014). Highly localized economies that have coalesced around the immediate needs of urban poor populations have reinforced existing structural inequalities such as intimate partner violence and gender discrimination. During a conversation with Mandla Majola, former district coordinator for the TAC in Khayelitsha, he noted his concerns about the correlation between the high incidence of rape and HIV infection in South Africa's poorest communities.

> Here [in Khayelitsha] rape is a very serious problem. We have three or four reported rape cases every day. Not per week, not per month, every day. And those are the cases that actually get reported. How many go unreported? No one can say for sure. There is no question that Khayelitsha's high AIDS statistics are the result of high levels of rape and sexual violence. (Interview with Mandla Majola, July 2014)

While no definitive explanation has been agreed upon, scholars have largely attributed these high levels of sexual violence, particularly rape, to historical trauma, what has become known as the "crisis of masculinity" (Reid and Walker 2005). Emerging from the dehumanization of Black men under apartheid, deindustrialization, and high levels of unemployment, some have argued that women's bodies became the target of these frustrations (Decoteau 2008). State-sponsored decentralization of industries such as textiles, paper, metals, and plastics, from urban to rural areas marked one of the first shifts in undermining established gender roles in South Africa. Women were more populous in the rural areas and the emergence of "industrial women" coupled with widespread male unemployment in the 1980s began to erode the largely male-dominated family structure (Hunter 2010).

As a result, women were beginning to wait longer before getting married and asserting themselves as independent social and economic entities. The presence of women in previously male gender roles further exacerbated the crisis of masculinity described by Decoteau (2008). Through what Kandirikirira (2002) refers to as "exaggerated masculinity" (119), disempowered South African men became increasingly aggressive within intimate relationships and sexually unaccountable. Self-worth and masculine identity became defined through having many lovers, many children, and demonstrable wealth. Thus, the erosion of social norms of masculinity in terms of material wealth, economic opportunities, and bride prices only served to strengthen an increasing trend of sexual violence.

This gradual, piecemeal societal transformation from historically patriarchal structures became ever more apparent in 1994 with the transition to majority rule, and in 1996 when the new South African constitution was approved by the constitutional court. As noted previously in this chapter, the postapartheid South African constitution is considered to be one of the most liberal in the world, and given the racist laws that preceded it, this is no real surprise. But in such a dramatic shift from the masculine heteronormativity of the apartheid state (Walker 2021b), to the progressive ideologies of the constitution, some areas of everyday life have been affected in unforeseen ways.

The transition to democracy radically changed prevailing social orders and catapulted the new nation into a modern and progressive state of being. As Decoteau (2013) argues, the new constitution's focus on rights was at times "problematically positioned in opposition to gendered 'traditions'" (166). Thus, the new ideologies espoused by the state often clashed radically with older and more conservative masculine values of South Africa's many cultures—as well as those of the apartheid state itself—and have shed light on extreme gender violence and oppression (Conway 2007; Hunter 2010; Decoteau 2013). Further, public debates about sexuality often problematically present a false dichotomy between "modernity" and "tradition," and typically culminate in what some scholars have referred to as the criminalization of tradition (Decoteau 2013).

That is to say, historical societal norms and values are often blamed for the high levels of sexual violence found in South Africa without adequately acknowledging the various economic and psychological impacts of extreme poverty, forced relocation, disempowerment, institutionalized racism, and other forms of structural violence.

Socially prescribed standards of masculinity may be undermined by poverty. Low or inconsistent incomes and/or unemployment may lead to an inability to meet socially and culturally constructed expectations of a male provider (Bhana and Pattman 2011). A powerful example of this can be found in the work of anthropologist Isaak Niehaus (2005). In his ethnography of sexual violence in the area of Bushbuckridge in rural Mpumalanga and interviews with self-identified rapists, many offenders were under the age of twenty-five and largely unable to meet the standards of masculinity expected of them in their community such as courting young women with gifts and other material romantic gestures. He notes that demonstrating masculinity was a foremost challenge, highlighting that "many young rapists were insecure and unable to assert their masculinity by other means" (Niehaus 2005, 72).

Moreover, low-income South African women also often demonstrate limited agency in their sexual debut and later experiences of sexual intimacy. When discussing their sexual experiences, some young Coloured women in the Western Cape intimated that they generally did not perceive their own apprehensiveness, discomfort, or pleasure as important considerations for their male partners, while acknowledging that such male dominance is largely fostered by disparities in equality and power within these relationships (Lesch and Kruger 2004). "Success" in masculinity, then, is purported to be situated in notions of wealth, social status, income, and power (Boonzaier 2005). Such perceived successes have been undermined by entrenched poverty, the restructuring of postapartheid South Africa's labor markets, and the country's developing discourses on women's rights.

While South Africa's sexual violence data are the most widely publicized, this is only the most visible aspect of widespread gender inequality from which numerous social HIV/AIDS risks can be traced. The importance placed upon a male's ability to provide material wealth to a potential intimate and/or romantic female partner, what has become known as provider masculinity (Hunter 2010), can help to account not only for the country's alarmingly high rape statistics but also for various forms of coercive or unequal sexual and intimate relationships. For South Africa's urban poor, sex and intimacy are often intertwined with gift-giving and the exchange of material goods, in which younger women are often propositioned by, usually older, men with disposable incomes (Hunter 2010; Aulette-Root, Boonzaier, and Aulette 2014). These relationships are distinct from transactional sexual relations found in sex work but maintain a number of the same problems, most notably that women involved in gift-giving relationships are often unable to enforce safe sex, further limiting their control of their own sexual health. Moreover, such gendered power imbalances embolden men to engage with multiple intimate partners. Young South African women are more likely to report serial monogamy, with relationships lasting from a few months to several years. However, men are more likely to report multiple concurrent sexual partners, with some data suggesting that men report concurrence at a rate three times higher than women (Karim 2010).

In a study on youth sexual relations in a KZN township, Bhana and Pattman (2011) found that "love is embedded in money, constructions of gender and not separate from sexual coercion and the pain of violence" (966). Gender norms in South Africa for girls may include social pressure to engage in high-risk sexual activity, early sexual debut, be in a relationship, or be submissive or passive (Cousins 2009). Gender norms for boys, however, are reflective of the aforementioned crisis of masculinity and may include social pressure to demonstrate sexual prowess, have multiple partners, provide material goods, and exercise control within those relationships (Cousins 2009). As a result, intimate relationships may bear the weight of physical violence, gender-based inequality, poor communication, and pressure to engage in high-risk sexual behaviors for HIV transmission. Intimate partner violence, conservative constructions of masculinity, inequalities at a personal and societal level, and sexual violence are some of the principal factors that militate against individual agency in sexual contact (Mswela 2009; Jewkes et al. 2010). For the nation's poor, South Africa has become a place in which romantic and sexual relationships shoulder the burdens of violent histories (Henderson 2011).

Alcoholism and substance abuse are further symptoms of structural violence that perpetuate high HIV/AIDS statistics and are common throughout South Africa's urban informal areas. While variations can be observed according to age, occupation, gender, and socioeconomic status, parts of the country exhibit high levels of alcoholism (Peltzer, Davids, and Njuho 2011). Alcohol abuse is most prevalent in Coloured communities, with binge drinking common among young urban males (Peltzer, Davids, and Njuho 2011). This has several implications for HIV prevention. Informal drinking establishments have been identified as increasing the probability of risky sexual encounters, and alcoholism has been associated with inconsistent condom use and domestic violence (Kalichman et al. 2008). Unprotected sex leads to a heightened risk of sexually transmitted infections (STIs), which in turn increases the chance of HIV transmission. This risk is far higher for women than it is for men.

Though scholars have noted that beers and spirits had been brewed in Africa long before European settlement, and in many sub-Saharan African cultures drinking alcohol is viewed as primarily a masculine social activity, this does not account fully for the unequal distribution of alcoholism among South Africa's poor (Mager 2010;). Structural factors, including the forced removals mentioned earlier in this chapter and the dehumanization of non-White South Africans under the apartheid regime, manufactured social problems within the country's most vulnerable populations. For psychologists Aulette-Root, Boonzaier, and Aulette (2014) the "structural changes that destroyed communities, jobs and homes, along with the psychological trauma of these changes and the removals themselves created new neighbourhoods with high levels of unemployment, crime, and alcohol and drug abuse" (20). This protracted and trans-generational psychological trauma has resulted in various crises of identity and masculinity that have manifested as some of the most urgent risks of HIV infection.

A Zebra Discussion? Coloured Communities, Historical Trauma, and the HIV/AIDS Crisis

In the discussion of the systematic disenfranchisement and marginalization of South Africa's population, it is important not to ignore the history of the country's Coloured communities and the impact of such social engineering within them. These communities, predominantly in the Western Cape, account for a significant amount of the province's low-income population. They represent a majority group in some of the largest townships surrounding Cape Town, known collectively as the Cape Flats. Coloured communities approached their racial discrimination differently from other South Africans, initially seeking a more moderate and assimilationist approach during the colonial period (Adhikari 2005). As a result, the political and economic effects that propel HIV/AIDS incidence within Coloured areas, while they bear many similarities, are not identical to those among other groups.

Perhaps the most substantial obstacle to any discussion of Coloured history is the dominance of European voices in articulating early encounters with South Africa's indigenous precolonial population and later records regarding slaves from Southeast Asia. Mindful of this, however, there is still benefit in examining the history through which the diverse cultural and ethnic groups that became known as "Coloured" were formed. In contrast to the term's use in the United States, in South Africa, "Coloured" does not refer to Black South Africans but rather a very broad collection of cultures and ethnicities that have developed over the centuries. In the early years of Dutch settlement in the Cape, the Khoikhoi and San peoples were often abducted during skirmishes by European militias and forced into slavery under the rising "Cape Gentry" (Dooling 2007). As the descendants of the Khoikhoi and San peoples, Cape slaves from South East Asia, Black and White South Africans, Coloured South Africans are generally regarded as of mixed heritage and have held an indeterminate status within the country's racial politics (Adhikari 2005). Coloured South Africans largely slipped through the cracks of the standard dichotomic narrative of White supremacy and Black subjugation. Despite their medial position—enjoying more rights than their Black compatriots but fewer rights than the White colonists—during British colonial rule, Coloured South Africans often continued to live in poverty and were subject to abuse and discrimination long after the abolition of slavery in 1808 (Aulette-Root, Boonzaier, and Aulette 2014).

While very much brutalized under apartheid, the attrition of Coloured rights was an altogether slower process than that of their Black compatriots. Where Black South Africans had been systematically discriminated against since the earliest European settlement, albeit informally, Coloured rights remained theoretically similar to those of Europeans in the Cape Colony under British colonial rule. The pace of erosion of Coloured liberties, however, quickened around the 1910 union with the eligibility of Coloured representatives in parliament being removed. Further laws in the 1920s and 1930s targeted Coloured education (Juvenile Affairs Act 1921, Apprenticeship Act 1922), and by the 1950s, Coloured South Africans were also being forcibly removed from cities, predominantly in the Cape, to government-prescribed "locations" (Adhikari 2005).

Adhikari (2005) notes that because "the primary objective was to assimilate into the dominant society, politicised Coloured people initially avoided forming separate political organisations" (4). One early and notable exception to this would be the creation of the African Political Organization—a political group that sought to improve the social and economic conditions of Coloured South Africans—in 1905. The organization largely attempted to influence the current order toward the benefit of its communities, rather than undermine it. The later policies of apartheid, however, discriminated with equal vigor against Coloured and Black South Africans. Despite this, the perception that Coloured political leaders and organizations negotiated within early racist governments as well as a complex relationship with cultural assimilation and creolization—which sociologist Zimitri Erasmus (2001) identifies as "the construction of an identity out of elements of ruling class as well as subaltern cultures" (16)—has left South Africa's Coloured communities in an unusual position within the country's political economy: not White enough for apartheid but not Black enough for the ANC. This in-between identity is perhaps most observably manifested in the postliberation era in the lack of economic opportunities, and at times the stripping of former opportunities from Coloured communities under the ANC's Black Economic Empowerment (BEE) initiative.

It is well-documented that the AIDS crisis has unfolded along racial lines, with Black South Africans bearing the brunt of new infections. However, despite similar population sizes, Coloured South African communities suffer a higher HIV/AIDS burden than their White compatriots (Walker 2022a). Moreover, similar determinants and symptoms of structural violence manifest within the country's Coloured communities. One of the more prominent issues is that of women's rights and gender inequality. Women in Coloured communities are subject to analogous forms of patriarchal social hierarchies found in many of South Africa's cultures (Aulette-Root, Boonzaier, and Aulette 2014). Coloured women, by occupying a lower status than that of men within an already marginalized demographic, are on the fringes of the fringe. Coloured women, as such, bear a similar burden of marginalization when compared to Black South Africans.

AIDS-Related Stigma and the Culture of Silence

Since HIV/AIDS was first discovered, it has been associated with fear, discrimination, misrepresentation, and blame. Characterizing the disease as an "epidemic of signification," Treichler (1987) highlighted the various meanings and judgments cultivated around the virus across the world. From

America's "gay plague" to South Africa's women's disease, the transferal of social responsibility for the virus onto the disempowered is a common and recurring theme (Decoteau 2008). This geography of blame (Farmer 1999) is often interwoven with structural inequalities and acute racism. In South Africa in particular, these forces collided with one another to develop into narratives of witchcraft, polluted bodies, and African sexualities as dangerous, uncontrolled, and promiscuous (McNeill 2011; Robins 2008).

In the early years of the HIV/AIDS epidemic, AIDS-related stigma presented a significant risk to the physical safety of PLHIV. A powerful example of this danger can be found in the story of AIDS activist Gugu Dlamini, who was brutally murdered in 1998 by members of her own community of KwaMashu, KwaZulu-Natal, after revealing her HIV status over the radio on World AIDS Day (Okigbo 2016). One of her killers justified the murder by claiming that Dlamini had brought shame to the community and degraded its reputation by associating it with the disease (Morrell 2003). While speaking out about HIV at this time was an extremely courageous act, this high-profile death did little to improve the safety for those with HIV, and violence against PLHIV persisted.

A less publicized but no less tragic murder of an AIDS activist occurred in 2003 in the Cape Town township of Khayelitsha. Lorna Mlosana was a twenty-one-year-old volunteer for the TAC when she was killed. Two men followed her to an outdoor toilet where they gang-raped her. A friend of Mlosana happened upon the incident and attempted to intervene. In the momentary lapse in violence, Mlosana disclosed that she was HIV-positive. The men brutally attacked the two women, leaving Mlosana dead and her friend severely injured. Stories such as these not only highlight the violence against PLHIV but also the fear, anger, and blame that have characterized representations of the illness.

With the rollout of ART, increasing numbers of South Africans were able to live healthier lives without the outward signifiers of illness. ART has the potential to reduce both internally and externally imposed stigma by diminishing associations between HIV/AIDS and death or disfigurement, and thus normalize the disease (Zuch and Lurie 2012; Peltzer and Ramlagan 2011). Despite achieving great strides in ART rollout since 2004, however, negative attitudes and opinions toward PLHIV in South Africa have remained stubbornly high. Recent research has highlighted the continued use of distancing and othering language to discuss issues related to HIV (Black 2019; Walker 2022a).

Social othering associated with AIDS coalesced with local cultural taboos around discussions of sex and death (McNeill 2011). Western Christian influences of purity and prudishness, which filtered into the collective consciousness from the early Christian missions, contributed to the emergence of a culture of silence around AIDS (Okyere-Manu 2013). Scholars have noted difficulties in communication between parents and children on the subject of sex in contemporary South Africa, which has been characterized as an "alarming failure of communication between parents and children on sexual issues" (Delius and Glaser 2002, 27) leading to poor awareness of safe sexual practices. Indeed, through surveys of young adults by students at the University of Cape Town, Levine and Ross (2002) found that very few respondents noted having gained their understanding of HIV and surrounding issues from their parents. Intergenerational taboos on discussing issues relating to sex served to reinforce prevailing norms of silence around HIV.

While stigma is a significant social obstacle for PLHIV, particularly those in close-knit communities where confidentiality in diagnoses may not be easily maintained (Walker 2022a), it is not experienced equally. Women, in particular, are acutely at risk of ostracization. Many South African men in the 1990s blamed young women's sexual promiscuity as the cause of the epidemic (Morrell 2003). As noted earlier, the incidence of gender-based violence has remained high, and socially constructed understandings of sexual violence as shameful—or at least not something to be openly discussed—has contributed to a climate in which this behavior can thrive. A further effect is that complications that are a consequence of sexual violence—such as psychological trauma, unwanted pregnancy, illegitimate abortions, and HIV infection—are concealed from public view, despite the very obvious physical and emotional effects on the victims.

Aulette, Boonzaier, and Aulette-Root (2014) note that "there are differences in regard to the extent to which men and women are blamed for their actions that supposedly led to their HIV-positive status" (43). Unequal social structures and the subordinate status of women within Black and Coloured communities further increase their risk of stigma and blame. They note that in societies in which masculine hegemony goes largely unchallenged, women are deemed less valuable, less intelligent, or weak if they conform to their gender role, and behaving improperly—often worthy of punishment—if they act outside of those formulae. Thus, not only are South African women more at risk of contracting the virus through various physiological and socioeconomic vulnerabilities but HIV-positive South African women from the hardest-hit communities are discriminated against twofold, and "HIV stigmatisation, therefore, adds to the 'normal' marginalisation of women" (2014, 43).

Finally, AIDS-related stigma exerts a negative influence on decisions to know one's HIV status, and thus begin treatment (Visser and Sipsma 2013). Hodes (2011) notes that even after the United States and Europe had reduced their AIDS mortality rates by 84 percent in the 1990s, South African advocates "were presented with the daunting task of reforming public opinion about HIV as a disease of shame and death when, for the majority of HIV-positive South Africans, this remained the stark reality" (159). In the face of such stigma, blame, and the silence that descended over the subject of AIDS in the early decades of the epidemic, reinforced by state-sponsored AIDS denial (which will be discussed later in this book), it is unsurprising then that early HIV campaigns in sub-Saharan Africa offered the opposite expression of making as much noise about HIV/AIDS as possible. In the wake of the murder of Gugu Dlamini, the TAC launched their Break the Silence campaign, a theme that was adopted by a number of organizations and peaked with the 46664 concerts between 2003 and 2008. The "shout" became the counterbalance to the culture of silence (Barz 2006).

Conclusion

South Africa's HIV/AIDS epidemic is as complex as it is widespread. Intricate and multifaceted, the story of AIDS in South Africa weaves together interconnected histories and narratives with roots that run deep into the country's colonial past. It is clear, as with many post-colonies, that the legacies of racial oppression live on in the structural violence experienced every day by many South Africans. Though impossible to summarize a full account of the epidemic that covers all its facets and historical and social determinants in the space available in one chapter, the purpose has been to highlight the fundamental historical context through which to understand the emergence of the world's most acute AIDS crisis.

While it would be considerably more straightforward to examine HIV/AIDS in strictly biomedical terms, ignoring the history, structural violence, and various determinants outlined above risks affirming the inevitability of the scale of the epidemic. Generations of violence have cultivated a social, political, and economic landscape in which an epidemic could rip through the poorest of South Africa's people. And while White minority rule may have ended, the specters of apartheid have continued to haunt postliberation South Africa.

Successive postapartheid governments' eagerness to implement neoliberal economic and social policies highlights the changing face of oppression. Within the poisonous cocktail of structural inequalities, entrenched poverty, sexual violence, and neoliberal policy, notions of human agency and individual choice become increasingly compromised.

3

Developing Durkheim

Musical Effervescence

The ethnographic vignettes scattered throughout these pages are designed to highlight something that I have found to be true of much human interaction involving music, that few other performative elements of our human condition are able to animate us more readily. Musical activities are, in the overwhelming majority of cases, participatory to some degree or another. Simultaneously, they draw from us a range of emotional responses. What is it about musical experiences that facilitates at the same time both the deeply personal and the fundamentally social? The ability of music to cultivate emotional resonance, bring humans together, and create connections between them sonically, physiologically, psychologically, and socially, forms the key to understanding the relationships between the multitude of applications of song within the South African AIDS crisis and their potential effectiveness toward social or health outcomes.

I noted in Chapter 1 that this book adopts an approach that reframes the seemingly disparate employment of song within the South African AIDS epidemic as manifestations of the same sets of phenomena operating through the same principles in different contexts and for different purposes. It is within this chapter that I elaborate upon that statement in full detail. It is quite likely that you have never come across the term that comprises part of the title of this chapter, "musical effervescence." For this reason, and that of clarity, it is perhaps best that I begin, admittedly bluntly, with some definitions to shed some light on this fairly uncommon collocation. Before I do so, however, it is important to acknowledge at this stage that there is no universally accepted definition of what music is or how it works. Indeed, some scholars contend that there are more definitions of music than there are cultures or subcultures throughout the world (Cook 1998), so any definitions constructed in these pages will continue to be subject to vigorous and animated debate. Nevertheless, tentative definitions are necessary to ground a framework in contemporary understandings of musical experiences.

Creating Connections: Collective Effervescence

First described by French sociologist Émile Durkheim in his work *The Elementary Forms of the Religious Life* ([1912] 2008), the term "collective effervescence" describes a phenomenon in which groups of individuals become physically, affectively, and emotionally animated through focused collective interaction rituals. He observed that when people come together in large groups and focus their collective attention, a type of intense and visceral "electricity" may be felt among them. That is to say, a form of human potential energy waiting to be catalyzed into a multitude of as-yet-unrealized forms. I find the physics analogy to be quite appropriate here, insofar as potential energy describes the energy held by an object (or body) in relation to other objects (or bodies) and is specifically influenced by the mass of, and distance between, those bodies. It also blends seamlessly with Durkheim's own metaphor of electricity that helps to explain not only the emotive and affective charge that permeates these assemblies but also the more primal and unmediated elements associated with the concentration of large numbers of individuals in one place. After all, electricity is powerful and extremely useful, but it has the potential to be wild, unpredictable, and even dangerous if left uninsulated or unmanaged.

While studying the ritual life of the indigenous communities of central Australia, Durkheim observed that individuals would experience heightened emotional and affective states of being through collective interpersonal interactions. The focus of attention (or what might be understood as the purpose of collective action) in these original examinations of collective effervescence was religious in nature, providing the impetus for highly animated and performative ritual processes. In these rituals, boundaries between individual and collective identity would become blurred as previously strict conventions governing social life temporarily fall away, allowing for the sharing of pleasures, taboos, ideals, and radical ideas. He notes that through collective effervescence it is possible to align the attitudes and opinions of those involved and increase susceptibility to suggestion.

> Every sentiment expressed finds a place without resistance in all the minds, which are very open to outside impressions; each re-echoes the others, and is re-echoed by the others. The initial impulse thus proceeds, growing as it goes, as an avalanche grows in its advance. And as such active passion so free from all control could not fail to burst out, on every side one sees nothing but violent gestures, cries, veritable howls, and deafening noises of every sort which aid in intensifying still more the state of mind which they manifest. ([1912] 2008, 215–16)

The act of connecting with others through assembling as a collective can not only stimulate a tendency toward collective thought and action (Shilling and Mellor 1998) but also further introduce and strengthen the potential for forms of action far beyond that which could be expected of individuals under regular conditions. This will become particularly relevant to understanding how people who were extremely ill marshaled enough energy to take part in physically demanding rallies and protests. Durkheim observed that those within an effervescent assembly appear to feel able to achieve the previously unachievable.

> In the midst of an assembly animated by a common passion, we become susceptible of acts and sentiments of which we were incapable when reduced to our own forces; and when the assembly is dissolved and when, finding ourselves alone again, we fall back to our ordinary level, we are then able to measure the height to which we have been raised above ourselves. (Durkheim [1912] 2008, 209–10)

While Durkheim focused his attention on the religious aspects of collective effervescence, the phenomenon is neither exclusive to religious proceedings nor to the indigenous Australians who first inspired him to develop his theory. To be sure, many religious events across the world may be described as exhibiting various degrees of effervescence, but many do not. Simultaneously, a number of contemporary secular events that involve large numbers of people congregating together have demonstrated a propensity for cultivating heightened emotional states among participants (consider protests, political rallies, riots, or sporting events).

Regardless of the catalyst, however, collective effervescence results in a significant increase in visceral and psychological stimulation, which in turn may fuel openness to new ideas (Olaveson 2001; Durkheim [1912] 2008). Effervescent assemblies are described as euphoric, outside of normal existence, and influenced by seemingly superhuman forces (Pickering 2001). Durkheim describes people who "believe themselves transported into an entirely different world from the one they have before their eyes" (Durkheim [1912] 2008, 226). This process strengthens and nourishes individual minds through intense collective emotion (Shilling and Mellor 1998). As Shilling and Mellor argue, "collective emotional revitalization also gives rise to new collective ideas, ideals, and values" (Shilling and Mellor 2001, 44). Within such quasi-transcendental states of being, it is unsurprising that beliefs in idealized conceptions of relationships between people and wider society are, at times, thought to be attainable.

Durkheim determines this to be a form of manic creativity that can manifest from periods of intense effervescence. He notes

> That general effervescence results which is characteristic of revolutionary or creative epochs. Now this greater activity results in a greater stimulation of individual forces. Men see more and differently than in normal times. Changes are not merely shades and degrees; men become different. The passions moving them are of such an intensity that they cannot be satisfied except by violent or unrestrained actions, actions of super-human heroism or of bloody barbarism. (Durkheim [1912] 2008, 210–11)

This manically creative force is found throughout our lives and shapes not only the truly exceptional moments of human history but also the everyday and mundane. Within this manic creativity, individuals are said to be transformed, and in their state of transcendence from their prior selves, they in turn transform the world around them. They attribute exceptional possibilities and ideal formulations of existence to the everyday, the sacred, and the profane. As Durkheim sees it, the formulation of an ideal world in the thoughts of those in the grip of collective effervescence is fundamentally a product of social life and the presence and proximity of focused bodies and minds.

Developing a Theory of Musical Effervescence

How do displays such as those described by Durkheim materialize? What are the mechanisms that drive their processes? Durkheim gave precedence to describing the manifestations of collective effervescence and its role in the development of religious sentiment. But while within his writing, such energetic displays would occur seemingly spontaneously and with little indication of their source, some potential clues can be found within Durkheim's ([1912] 2008) own words.

> And since a collective sentiment cannot express itself collectively except on the condition of overserving a certain order permitting co-operation and movements in unison, these gestures and cries naturally tend to become rhythmic and regular; hence come songs and dances. (216)

* * *

> Commencing at nightfall, all sorts of procession, dances and songs had taken place by torchlight; the general effervescence was constantly increasing. (218)

* * *

> A man is carried outside himself and diverted from his ordinary occupation and preoccupations. Thus the same manifestations are to be observed in each case: cries, songs, music, violent movements, dances, the search for excitants that raise the vital level, etc. (383)

* * *

> If we set aside the funeral rites—the sombre side of every religion—we find the totemic cult celebrated in the midst of songs, dances, and dramatic representations. (224)

In these excerpts, Durkheim notes that songs, music, and vocalizations were present as the effervescent assemblies were developing. The sonorous and rhythmic elements of music are interwoven within Durkheim's outline of effervescence, but where he describes song, dance, and rhythmic chant as products of an effervescent assembly, I argue that they can be, and often are, fundamental components in its creation and maintenance.

Building upon the foundation of collective effervescence, a theory of musical effervescence can be cultivated to account for the heightened affective states of being associated with groups involved in participatory musicking toward specific goals, beliefs, or purposes. I argue that musical effervescence manifests through the culmination of several factors including (1) purpose, (2) participatory musicking with others, (3) synchronicity, and (4) heightened affective states of being that manifest in (5) Durkheim's manic creativity related to the initial purpose. Throughout the rest of this chapter, far from Durkheim's order permitting cooperation, I outline how the processes that culminate in musical effervescence draw from some of the earliest developments of our evolution and speak to the very heart of what it means to be human.

Participation

Music is a highly participatory medium of expression. This may seem obvious to most of us, particularly those who play in ensembles, dance, frequent nightclubs, or have just enjoyed a moment of shared interest with others upon passing a particularly engaging street performer. But the simplicity of this statement belies its fundamental importance to understanding the ways in which music is able to harness humans and bind us into shared space and time. One notable approach to the topic of participation comes from ethnomusicologist Thomas Turino (2008), who suggests that the power and importance of music lies predominantly in its tendency toward social cohesion. He points out that in many forms of music-making across the world, participation takes priority over perceived skill. Connections created through musical activities with others can strengthen feelings of belonging, shared identity, and social comfort that are some of the foundational aspects of the human experience. It is the social relations realized within these musical practices that are at the forefront of importance, rather than the production of an art form from which those social relations may be abstracted. A natural progression from this train of thought is to reposition participatory musical experiences at the core of the social life of humans and not, as many in the postindustrial West have come to believe, subservient to the serious business of professional musicians creating art and presentational performances.

Turino posits the idea of "sameness" through musical performance. That is to say, music is, at times, able to bond its participants together. Group musical performance may create spaces in which people transcend individual superficial differences such as class, gender, age, or race, and instead focus on shared commonalities. This model of sameness seems to draw influence from anthropologist Victor Turner's (1969) concept of communitas. For Turner, communitas describes periods of social equality among community members, through which regular social hierarchies are temporarily suspended and replaced by what he refers to as anti-structure, a state of unstructured society governed by commonality and solidarity over social stratification. He describes this as the process of "giving recognition to an essential and generic human bond, without which there could be *no* society" (97). Communitas is usually engendered through ritual processes or rites of passage and these events are often community-wide and co-performed, potentially drawing from a wide variety of performance media, including music.

Participatory musical events such as those described by Turner can provide the stimulus for proximity with others and the sharing of focus and purpose across a community. These elements can be the kindling from which musical effervescence erupts as they combine within a performance space to bind individuals together and encourage the kinds of manic creativity outlined by Durkheim—social relationships broken down into anti-structure only to be rebuilt as the ideals of the collective coalesce into social manifestations again once the ritual has ended. Turino's repackaging of communitas illustrates his view that musical activities have the potential to fundamentally alter the regular state of being among those involved. Indeed, whether in HIV/AIDS awareness and prevention musical theater shows or TAC rallies and protests, a foundational principle of this book is the capacity for music, in this case song, to be applied in ways that can and do change societies and lives.

Just as Turino does, it is not uncommon for theorists to draw from multiple disciplines in order to try to understand the complexities of the social aspects of music. In the hypothetical and byzantine Venn diagram of human life, music would likely appear within most of the circles. Recent attempts by sociologists, musicologists, and ethnomusicologists to unravel the purposes, functions, and raison d'être of music within society have turned to the earlier work of anthropologists such as Gregory Bateson (1972) and Edward Hall (1976) (see Small 1998; Turino 2008; Hesmondhalgh 2013). This is in large part due to the social and communicative properties of distinctly musical phenomena such as rhythm and pitch outlined by the two anthropologists.

Bateson's (1972) approach to the arts is one that suggests they are communicative media distinct from, but of equal importance to, spoken language. He notes that the arts form part of a communicative nexus that functions to integrate individuals into wider social groups. If identities are created, maintained, and modified in relation to others, whether within our social groups or outside of them, and these social relationships are perhaps some of the most primal of biological impulses, then our behavior may be profoundly influenced by the parts of this communicative nexus that are proto-lingual, concerned with gesture, patterns, and embodiment. As a matter of heuristics, scholars concerned with the evolution of human cognition overwhelmingly agree that the processes that guide organisms and species toward success do not easily tolerate activities that expend time and energy, as making music does while returning no material or social benefits to continued existence (Dunbar 2012). Moreover, notwithstanding the unwillingness of evolutionary processes to countenance such reckless profligacy, we might also note that if spoken language were sufficient to communicate every aspect of human existence—even accounting for Harvard linguist Steven Pinker's (1997) now notorious comments discounting music as nothing more than auditory cheesecake—then the music-making that we continue to find across the world would have disappeared long ago (Turino 2008).

For Hall (1976), synchronization forms a fundamental part of nonverbal communication. He notes that "being in sync is itself a form of communication" (71), insofar as it signals connectedness with others. Indeed, the natural state for human interpersonal relationships is one in which communicative (nonverbal or otherwise) parties become synchronically bound to one another's bodily micro-expressions and gestures. Moreover, rhythm, volume, and synchronization are also intimately linked in speech (Ludden 2016; Becker 2011). When engaged in conversation, speakers will often match each other's rhythmic tendencies and volume in both sonic and embodied ways. So fundamental to human communication is synchronicity with others, that to be out of sync is an inherently disruptive act. This is what makes delays in telephone calls so distracting (Black 2019) and one would likely find the experience of attempting to communicate with someone using vastly different speech speed or volume quite unsettling.

While enthusiasm for universal approaches to music has ebbed and flowed for much of the twentieth century, if Hall's theorizations are correct, then there may indeed be something universal about musical communication. As celebrated ethnomusicologist Bruno Nettl (2015) puts it, as the discipline sought to differentiate itself from more established areas of music studies, ethnomusicologists—while not necessarily incorrect in their assumptions or assessments—may have overstated the non-universality of how we experience music. Certainly, there is a recently emerging body of evidence, through collaborations across disciplines such as biology, psychology, and anthropology, that appears to indicate some potentially universally identifiable traits of music (Athanasopoulos et al. 2021; Yurdum et al. 2023; Ravignani, Delgado, and Simon Kirby 2017). Given that music unfolds over time and often in somewhat predictable patterns, such universality may be found in its ability to structure embodiment more forcefully than many other performing arts, providing an ideal conduit for embodied effervescence (DeNora 2013). The importance of music as a communicative tool can be found in the way it is able to create places, both spatially and temporally, for intimate and emotive alignment, social interconnectedness, shared spatial and temporal coordination, and embodiment of values or ideals (DeNora 2013).

Musicking

So fundamental to the social functions of music is the concept of participation that most ethnomusicological perspectives completely reject dichotomous conceptions of musical performer and listener, and instead prefer the more egalitarian concept of musicking (Small 1998). First introduced by Christopher Small in *Music of the Common Tongue* (1987) and then later refined in *Musicking* (1998), the concept of musicking outlines an approach to music that is inclusive of all musical experiences, regardless of ability or intent. The central idea is that music is not something to be considered abstractly or divorced from its social context. Instead, the lexical transformation of music (noun) to musicking (verb) necessitates the reconsideration of performance in terms of human encounters and experiences, that is to say, participation.

This approach describes musical experiences, regardless of how one contributes, as fundamentally human acts that do not discriminate based on so-called musical ability. For Small, then, everyone can music. Drawing from the work of early ethnomusicologists who conceptualized music not simply through its sonorous qualities but through its social functions (Merriam 1964; Blacking 1974), Small determined that musicking provides us with a vessel through which to model social relationships by way of the interconnectedness of musical experiences. Through musicking then, the most inwardly desired social relationships are made public and brought into existence for the duration of the musical event. The striking similarities between Small's musicking and Durkheim's observations of collectivized manic creativity and ideal conceptions of social life described earlier in this chapter seem to indicate that musical activities share a similar capacity to influence bodies and minds as the mass gatherings noted in *The Elementary Forms of the Religious Life*.

Many musical experiences are rituals of sorts, and the business of rituals is to affirm, explore, or celebrate individual and collective identities as they relate to each other or wider society. This sense of interconnectedness with others and shared identity within musical experiences is an important component in the socially cohesive properties of music. Across the world, participatory musical expressions are often the primary methods of expressive cultural practices through which people articulate shared and/or individual identities (Turino 2008).

But while the principle of musicking is an important component to the discussions in this book—particularly as they relate to the ways in which collective musical experiences are or are not able to cultivate the kinds of manic creativity noted earlier—a number of Small's points are ambiguous and limited in scope. It is unclear, for example, how including distinctly unmusical acts (both productive and receptive) within the concept of musicking contributes to a deeper understanding of musical experience. As a point of contact, Small argues that musicking as a phenomenon must be inclusive of, for example, those who are involved in setting up a performance space but are not involved in the performance in any further capacity thereafter. This exaggerated inclusivity dilutes the concept's otherwise important observations that it is music's social, experiential, connective, emotive, and affective qualities that afford it such ubiquity in human social life.

Despite this, the concept of musicking throws open the definition of what we might consider a musical activity. This book understands the concept of musicking in an inclusive but non-exaggerated way. To music is to take part in a musical experience in any capacity. The important distinction here is the formulation of a musical experience fundamentally as one that involves some direct contact with the sonorous aspects of music or others who are musicking. It reframes music from something we listen to, play, visually represent in scores, buy, sell, or own, to something that incorporates the entire act of performance, including people (performing or listening), places, actions, and relationships.

While the conception of music as a dynamic and inclusive process is interesting in its own right, it has further implications for this discussion of musical effervescence insofar as it offers a channel into understanding participatory behavior mediated by musical experience. Describing musicking, Small argues

> in making no distinction between what the performers are doing and what the rest of those present are doing, it reminds us that musicking [. . .] is an activity in which all those present are involved and for whose nature and quality, success or failure, everyone present bears some responsibility. (Small 1998, 10)

For Small, then, musicking describes a collective activity. While musicking may take any number of forms, it is those most immediately participatory forms that are often the most socially cohesive (Turino 2008). Given that much of the world's music is not primarily predicated on accuracy, virtuosity, or compositional intent but on the level of participation and musicking from those involved, it is reasonable to conclude that, for the vast majority of the world, music is a social phenomenon. By moving synchronously, it is possible to experience a connection with others. Durkheim ([1912] 2008) noted this phenomenon during his observations of the creative and idealized conceptions of the world, in the manic creativity noted earlier. While Small (1998) does not use the same sort of evocative language as Durkheim, similar principles can be found within musicking, describing the phenomenon as a way of modeling "ideal relationships as the participants imagine them to be" (13), in terms of both person-to-person interaction but also interaction between the individual and the wider society.

Synchronicity and Entrainment

The vocabulary commonly used by anthropologists to describe everyday life exudes musicality. John Blacking speaks of the *rhythm* of culture and the *cycles* of human life in terms of seasonal change, physical growth, economic development and so forth (Blacking, Byron, and Nettl 1995). Given that music is able to structure inchoate bodies into shared space and time (DeNora 2013), a strong case can be made that it presents a unique vehicle for creative and expressive communication. As noted earlier, musical experiences often manifest in the form of ritualistic behaviors through which humans explore and communicate identities, experience and express emotions, and interact with other humans in physical and embodied ways. Fundamental to such interaction rituals are the mechanisms through which people become synchronized in one another's physical micro-rhythms and emotions (Hall 1976; von Scheve 2012; Walker 2021a).

Drawing inspiration from the Dutch physicist Christiaan Huygens, who discovered the propensity of two independently oscillating pendulums to sympathetically synchronize when swung from the same board, the sub-discipline of biomusicology has theorized similar forms of synchronicity among humans, postulating shared musical experiences as the coupling factor in the form of entrainment. This describes "a process whereby two rhythmic processes interact with each other in such a way that they adjust towards and eventually 'lock in' to a common phase and/or periodicity" (Clayton, Sager, and Will 2004, 2). Not only does it have interesting implications for the synchronization of humans by way of external rhythmic stimuli such as music, it also presents a unique way of understanding those stimuli. Entrainment through musicking suggests that musical activities are rendered meaningful not only through the decoding of aural or sonorous properties, but also are interpreted, expressed, and understood in embodied ways (Clayton, Sager, and Will 2004), similar to the synchronicity in communication described by Hall (1976).

There are numerous examples of physical and psychological entrainment discussed across a number of disciplines including fireflies illuminating in synchrony (Wilson and Cook 2016), shared speech rhythms (Cummins 2009), and various synchronizations of physiological cycles among groups of people (Roenneberg and Merrow 2007). But while entrainment as a concept may be used to describe measurable and observable phenomena, the processes that result in the synchronization of systems are as varied as their examples. Put simply, entrainment describes the outcomes of processes not the processes themselves. With this in mind, it is important to look closely at the particular set of processes that culminate in the entrainment of individuals through music and how they may be understood within musical effervescence.

If each individual human is considered to have multiple physiological and cognitive oscillations, then entrainment through music would be the result of the process of aligning those oscillations through an external musical stimulus. This can be achieved through musical meter, rhythm, or pulse (Large and Kolen 1994; Eck, Gasser, and Port 2000; Thaut, McIntosh, and Hoemberg 2015). Indeed, recent research has suggested that beat induction—that is the ability not only to anticipate a beat but to instinctively evaluate which beats are more prominent within a rhythmic pattern—is observable among newly born infants, strongly indicating that the interpretation and anticipation of rhythm is innate among humans (Honing et al. 2009; Winkler et al. 2009). This would certainly support Hall's position that synchronicity is a fundamental component within the social lives of humans. And further, that it is only through habituation with one's own cultural forms of gesture and communication that we gradually lose the ability to tap into the embodied micro-rhythms of all human forms of communication.

When considering entrainment through musicking, one might naturally gravitate toward a mental image of groups of people dancing together to the same beat. While this is a valid representation of synchronicity, recent studies have begun to unpack significantly less immediately observable and more complex ways in which music may entrain our bodies and minds. Neurologists have found that various neural oscillations in the parts of the brain associated with the recognition and interpretation of auditory stimuli respond to and entrain with meter and frequency of musical stimuli (Stephan et al. 2002; Grahn, Henry, and McAuley. 2011; Thaut, McIntosh, and Hoemberg 2015). The entrainment of neurological oscillations has significant implications in the field of clinical music therapy. But perhaps less immediate but equally important implications relate to our understanding of the potentially profound effect of music on the minds, emotions, and psychological processes of those who are musically entrained and the influence it may have on experiences of social interconnectedness through musical synchronization.

While a relative newcomer to the discussion of interpersonal experiences in music, the concept of "social entrainment" has been around since the late twentieth century. The term was coined by McGrath and Kelly (1986) to describe the synchronization of human psychological and physiological rhythms to external pacers and social cues. The fact that entrainment has only recently been applied to the practice of music has been a significant oversight in music scholarship, given that the social aspects of musicking are fundamentally built upon interconnections with others. That is to say that musicking experiences, given their overwhelmingly social and communicative properties, draw heavily from the social bonding of entrained bodies.

When bodies are entrained through musicking, they not only share time and space but the embodiment of that communality culminates in synchronized physiological, neurological, and psychological processes, perhaps leading to the propensity for agreement among the effervescent assemblies described by Durkheim. Indeed, there is some evidence to suggest that moving together in time with another person blurs the perception of self and others (Overy and Molnar-Szakacs 2009), and shared psychological experiences within collective activities have been observed by early sociological studies of crowd behavior (Durkheim [1912] 2008). Through creating what Turino (2008) refers to as "social intimacy" (3) by way of participatory musical experience, emotions, feelings, and affective states associated with the musical event are often felt to be innate or true. This raises questions regarding the biological mechanisms through which participating in musicking experiences may influence thoughts and behaviors.

"Musilanguage" and the Evolution of the Musical Brain

Musicking affects every part of our body, from a molecular level to the most complex tissues of our brain (Schneck and Burger 2006). It is our entire bodies that interpret acoustic vibrations, not just our auditory sensory apparatus, and the conscious mind is only cognizant of the extent of the body's response in a limited capacity. Indeed, musicking is often a deeply enjoyable experience, physically altering the neurochemistry of our brains.

Some scholars have argued that it is not enough to base the ubiquity of music in human life exclusively on the pleasurable aspects of musicking (see Turino 2008). While there is merit to this caution, there is a wealth of evidence that indicates that the temporal structures of musicking that communalize both space and time are often embodied by the individuals themselves, and a plethora of biopsychosocial rewards are achieved through the successful participation. Even listening to music without any additional stimuli has been shown to release mood-regulating endorphins (Moraes et al. 2018), with sports scientists associating listening to music with increased levels of dopamine during exercise, resulting in improvements in athletic performance (Sutoo and Akiyama 2004).

As the central processer of all this sensory data, the activity of the brain, whether we are conscious of it or not, can be significantly influenced by this sensory input. Evidence that the social importance of music is built into our physiology can be found within brain neurochemistry and the influence of musical stimuli on various hormones that regulate human behavior. For example, Campbell, Ophir, and Phelps. (2009) found that raising or lowering the level of oxytocin, a hormone strongly associated with social bonding, reproduction, and mother-child connections in the weeks after childbirth, in the brains of certain species of mice that are known for their complex socialized vocalizations had profound effects on their ability to develop and maintain connections with other individuals. Other researchers have found that vocalizations increased with the artificial introduction of the hormone, while those with reduced levels demonstrated fewer vocalizations, abnormal behavior, and increased stress responses (Floody, Cooper, and Albers 1998). While these studies were conducted on particular species of highly social rodents, recent studies have associated activities such as maternal speech around infants, singing lessons among adults, and low-volume music during open-heart surgery to increased levels of oxytocin in humans (Seltzer, Ziegler, and Pollak 2010; Nilsson 2009; Grape et al. 2003), perhaps suggesting similar associations between the social bonding hormone and musicking among humans.

Musicking together also appears to influence our ability to respond empathically with others, further associating it with the social aspects of human existence. Of the kinds of empathy displayed by humans, emotional or affective empathy is concerned with assessing and understanding the emotions of others, while self-reflective empathy relates to our capacity to view a situation from the perspective of someone else. Both of these forms of empathy are supported by different parts of the brain that are recruited so that we are able to feel vicariously the emotional and physical pain and pleasures of others. What is striking is the extent to which these regions of the brain spring to life when engaging in musicking activities (Harvey 2017). The significant musical-empathic overlaps in the geographies of the brain associated with social cooperation, altruism, and belonging strongly indicate that the social importance of music is an evolutionary adaptation and a biological determinant of modern human behavior.

That our brains appear to be hardwired to connect socially and empathically with one another through musical pathways becomes clearer when considering the possible ancient roots of musicking within human prehistory and evolution. While debated within paleo-linguistic, archaeological, and paleo-musicological circles, some scholars maintain that the ability to phonologically rearrange and organize sounds is a necessary prerequisite to language (Marler 2000). Others still argue that music is as old, if not older, than what might be described as early spoken language (Dunbar 2017).

Discourses on the origins of music are numerous and interdisciplinary, but there are two main themes that divide the literature. The first connects bipedalism, our ability to walk on two legs, to rhythm and synchronicity. As noted earlier in this chapter, synchronization provides avenues through which modern humans may create and strengthen interpersonal connections. This relationship between social bonding and entrainment through the rhythm of footfall may have helped to strengthen social bonds between early humans. While no definitive explanation can be provided for our ancestors' transition to bipedalism, the most convincing evidence we have to date involves two stages. The first stage involves the emergence of a partial upright gait among the early australopithecines of sub-Saharan Africa, which developed into the full bipedal anatomy of *Homo ergaster* in the second stage, around one million years later (Mithen 2005).

One of the more persuasive theories to explain the partial bipedalism of the australopithecines comes from observations of modern chimpanzees. Hunt (1994) notes in a detailed study of chimpanzee behavior that their use of a bipedal gait was primarily reserved for gathering low-hanging fruit from small trees. He observed that when moving from one tree to the next, instead of returning to their typical knuckle-walking form of locomotion, the animals would remain upright and waddle the short distances from one tree to the next. This form of elementary bipedalism not only allows the chimpanzees to use both hands when collecting fruit but also avoids unnecessary energy expenditures relating to postural changes (Mithen 2005; Hunt 1994). Anatomical characteristics more suited to standing rather than extended bipedal walking found in fossilized australopithecine remains strengthen the extrapolation of these observations to suggest that early hominids may have behaved in similar fashions. This temporary bipedalism may have engendered specific rhythmic movements over time, eventually leading to a certain degree of synchronization among small groups of hominids.

Modern humans have been shown to have a tendency for synchronizing step periodicity and speed when walking together, despite the influence of potentially disruptive variables such as leg length or gait idiosyncrasies (Nessler and Gilliland 2009; Zivotofsky and Hausdorff 2007; Nessler et al. 2013). In doing so, one might suggest that such an innate propensity for entrainment may have significant effects on interpersonal relationships in social groups. Indeed, Nagasaka et al., (2013) have noted that spontaneous social synchronization among Japanese macaques produces positive social interactions in lab settings, indicating that the phenomenon of synchronization may be socially rewarding, not just for humans, but also for other primates.

While humans are not the only animals to have developed bipedal locomotion, we are the only primate to consistently utilize this method of movement. The anatomically modern human gait involves rhythmic consistencies across variables including speed, stride duration, and stride length (Terrier, Turner and Schutz 2005; Larsson, Richter, and Ravignani 2019). The average frequency of human footfall tends to be within the range of around 75 and 125 steps per minute, closely resembling the average beats per minute found in much of the world's music. While this may be coincidental, researchers are beginning to connect our current musical outputs, particularly those focused primarily on physical bodily participation such as dancing, with our capacities for rhythmic embodied participation as a result of our bipedal step frequency (Leman et al. 2013; Styns et al. 2007; Changizi 2011).

The second theme connects the development of language with the development of musicking to some common ancestor that predates both. The term "musilanguage" has been popularized by evolutionary psychologist and anthropologist Steven Brown (2000, 2017) to describe this theory. It is perhaps impossible to know the point in prehistory that may be identified as the moment we began to speak (such is the nature of evolution that it is presumed to have developed incrementally over time), but most agree that spoken language may be traced to anatomically modern *Homo sapiens* in Southern Africa around 150,000 to 200,000 years ago (Fleagle et al. 2008; Poznik et al. 2013; Pagel 2017).

The emergence of language is a significant turning point in human cultural evolution. Given the importance of language both within the story of humanity's development and our current existence (Harvey 2017), if forms of proto-lingual vocalizations are indeed the foundation of both language and music, then it would stand to reason that exploring the development of music from our ancient ancestors would be of equal importance to understanding ourselves as we are today. Scholars, however, only tentatively began to take this seemingly logical step in the 1980s and 1990s with the establishment of subdisciplines such as musical archaeology and evolutionary musicology.

Brown (2017) argues that the most convincing progenitor to spoken language must involve the expression of emotion. While emotion is discussed within the two main approaches to the emergence of human language—gestural and vocal theories—it is more commonly associated with vocalizations, as will be discussed later in this chapter. Gestural theories are the most recent development in this field and proponents of this approach suggest that communication among early humans may have developed first as a series of gestures used to articulate the basic aspects of everyday life such as spatial properties, objects, or actions (Armstrong and Wilcox 2007). Once again, it is bipedalism that is credited with the evolution of such communication, as walking upright freed our hands so that they may be used for other purposes (Gillespie-Lynch et al. 2013). While there may potentially be some interesting connections between gestural communication as a result of early bipedalism and the development of music, theories from this school of thought so far have had little to say on the matter.

Vocal approaches to the development of language have a much longer history than gestural theories, spanning as far back as Renaissance Europe and including works by French philosophers Étienne Bonnot de Condillac ([1746] 1971) and Jean-Jacques Rousseau ([1781] 1986). At the time, it would not have been uncommon to hear, for example, discussions around the communication of emotion within language and music, and the potential relationship between the two forms of human expression. More recently, the focus of vocal theories has shifted toward evolutionary innovations of speech such as adaptations in the human larynx and oral articulatory apparatus that could have made possible new syllable structures or phonemic repertoires (Brown 2017). However, a number of scholars argue that language and emotion co-evolved, with the production of specific vocalizations developing alongside our need to express these new feelings. Perspectives from evolutionary biology postulate that open-ended brain plasticity may have helped to reorganize existing brain tissue and neural structures in response to environmental or social stressors, such as increasingly complex cultures, that produced novel adaptive behaviors (West-Eberhard 2003; Jablonka, Ginsburg, and Dor 2012). Indeed, the emotional associations of music have also been speculated to be linked with the evolution of the basic emotional systems of the brain, given that some of our most primal emotions are characterized by distinct sounds in many mammalian species such as the lilting tones of joy, low guttural expressions of despair, or the soft articulations of maternal care (Panksepp 2009).

Brown (2017) notes that a musilanguage progenitor of both music and speech is likely to have developed from group choruses, not unlike those found among modern wolves or chimpanzees. It is probable that such choruses would have played a number of social functions in the community, including emotional articulations and group bonding. This has been discussed in what has become known as the "vocal grooming" hypothesis, in which vocalizations such as laughter and singing gradually replaced physical grooming as the primary method of creating and maintaining social bonds within ever-expanding bands of early humans (Dunbar 2017). These collectivized group vocalizations may have become increasingly ritualized within the communities. In doing so, meanings may have emerged around specific vocalizations that the entire collective would have been aware of and involved in, thus laying the foundation for the expression of emotive meanings through sound. At this stage, music and language would not yet have developed separate identities or purposes. It is likely that some intermediary step between this early musilanguage and verbal communication would have emerged to distinguish music from speech, perhaps not dissimilar to a group-level grammelot, that is to say, a fictitious set of vocalizations that utilize the prosodic elements of language while composed of ad hoc phonetic gibberish (Jaffe-Berg 2001).

While such theories are difficult, perhaps sometimes impossible to prove, they illustrate that there is a growing chorus (pun intended) of academics and researchers that reject Pinker's auditory cheesecake and the implications it presents for musicking in human life. Indeed, even Darwin expended considerable energy contemplating the roles of music within human evolution, though he was often perplexed by its universality. For example, he notes in *The Descent of Man* (1871), that it is probable that early humans would have used pre-lingual vocalizations in a similar manner to modern gibbons to attract mates and increase social harmony. While ultimately a simplistic view of early musicking, Darwin may not have been wrong about it. Musicking is an extremely pro-social behavior and publicly shared expressive culture are some of the most fundamental ways through which modern humans create and maintain social groups and identities, which are, as Turino (2008) notes, essential to survival.

Musicking, in its most primal forms, may have developed alongside our progressively complex social interconnectedness, perhaps not exclusively as a result of our evolving cognitive abilities but rather in tandem with them. Studies have recently begun to determine associations between high levels of social behavior and trends toward cortical expansion (Dunbar 1996, 2003; Barton 2006; Dunbar and Shultz 2007; Schulkin and Raglan 2014). It is postulated that the pressures of coming into contact with others, managing relationships, and creating and tracking alliances require more cortical mass which resulted in this expansion (Schulkin and Raglan 2014). The social cognitive skills required to regulate ever more complex social structures may have developed alongside our increasing use of musilanguage vocalizations to maintain social harmony. If social cohesion has been fundamental to our survival as a species, and participatory musically expressive experiences have provided a central component in maintaining these social connections, then taken to its logical conclusion, we can quite reasonably infer that musicking has been instrumental in the survival and eventual flourishing of the human species.

Music, Emotion, and Affect

Within the current elucidation of a theory of musical effervescence, this chapter has so far discussed the profound effects of participation and synchronization in creating short- and long-term bonds between humans as well as some of the possible biological and evolutionary processes that support them. It has yet to consider, however, the more animating features of musicking, the kind most readily associated with collective effervescence. Brown's (2017) calculation that the early musilanguage of pre-lingual hominids must have involved the expression of emotions speaks to one of the core elements of musical effervescence: music makes us feel things. Perhaps more than any other performing or creative art form, music is able to stir the passions of humans in ways that we still do not fully understand. This is certainly not through lack of trying. The story of our journey to demystify the links between music and emotion has spanned thousands of years. In ancient Greece, Plato (1980) noted that "more than anything else rhythm and harmony find their way to the inmost soul and take strongest hold on it" (664). While in ancient China, Confucius (2012) determined that "Music is that which moves man from the internal; rites are that which affects man on the external. Music brings about harmony. Rites ensure obedience" (125). In the millennia that have followed, contemplating the emotive power of music has proved to be a fascinating yet illusive pursuit.

The implications of the, admittedly hotly contested, universal language approach to music are that musical meanings transcend ordinary linguistic limitations and instead communicate through emotive and affective means, speaking fundamentally to a shared humanity in all of us (Nettl 2000). At the outset of this chapter, I posed a question concerning the intimacy and sociality of musical experiences, namely to do with how musicking is often able to be deeply personal while simultaneously social and connective. A discussion of the emotive nature of music may provide some insight into how these seemingly mutually exclusive properties may coexist. In actuality, these two properties necessitate one another.

While emotion has readily been associated with music for millennia, exploration of musicking's affective properties is relatively new. While it does not have the same illustrious history, it is worth discussing the phenomena this term can describe in order to theorize the often ineffable and indescribable effects of musicking. Indeed, the synchronization of thought outlined by Durkheim and Small implies a significant connection between entrainment of the physical body and entrainment of the mind. Furthermore, the kinds of affective responses described throughout the descriptions of the indigenous Australian rituals, while of course not articulated with the same terminology, are predicated on the rejection of the mind-body duality.

Affect may be thought of as describing the bodily experience of emotions, an implicitly holistic psycho-physiological phenomenon, and is often discussed in relation to our interaction with stimuli, whether human or otherwise. Unlike feelings or emotions, which are largely well-defined and easily described, affect can be experienced as entirely nebulous states of being and thus is one of our more detailed means of describing those experiences elicited through musicking, collective effervescence, or individual and mediated musical exposure such as through recorded music or music videos.

The affective turn in sociological writing in recent years has signaled renewed attention toward sensorial experiences that is of particular interest to scholars of the performing arts, as a result of what sociologists Hurley and Warner (2012) refer to as their "bodily entanglements in their production and sensate lures in their reception" (99). The turn toward affect represents a scholarly desire to understand the parts of human behavior that are not fueled by rational or cognitive processes but rather preconscious behavior and attitudes that are molded by social and cultural conventions.

Insofar as it is possible to define affect, Gregg and Seigworth offer the following tentative definition:

> Affect, at its most anthropomorphic, is the name we give to those forces—visceral forces beneath, alongside, or generally *other than* conscious knowing, vital forces insisting beyond emotion—that can serve to drive us toward movement, towards thought and extension, that can likewise suspend us (as if in neutral) across a barely registering accretion of force-relations, or that can leave us overwhelmed by the world's apparent intractability. (2010, 1)

These visceral responses may be familiar to anyone who has ever had goose bumps from listening to music or has ever been moved to tears by a particularly emotive scene in a movie (try watching it again without the accompanying film score to get a sense of how important music is to this phenomenon). Given the nebulous states of emotional stimulation created by music, affect becomes a fundamental conceptual component in understanding the mechanisms through which musical effervescence is able to animate and influence individuals and communities. Are those individuals aware that their thoughts, feelings, and opinions may change in affectively charged group settings as Durkheim described, at least in those moments? Are the individuals of an effervescent assembly cognizant of the influence of the collective on their perceptions, conceptions, and formulations of life and the world around them in their everyday and ideal forms? If not, then questions may be raised about how and why this seems to occur. Equally, if so, even more questions arise about why the phenomenon occurs regardless of the participants' awareness of the process.

Affect is often observed in response to some external force, but these external influences need not be forceful at all. Psychologists Gregg and Seigworth (2010) note that affect tends to occur or transpire "within and across the subtlest of shuttling intensities: all the minuscule or molecular events of the unnoticed" (2). Affective responses are likely to result from ill-defined affective moments or innocuous affective cues, perhaps phenomena which are so ubiquitous that they often go unseen or unheard. Affect displays, conscious or otherwise, can outwardly indicate affective processes among individuals or groups, oftentimes in physical manifestations, perhaps through specific behaviors like dancing (or unintentional movement to music such as foot-tapping), facial expressions, or other gestures. These visceral responses represent a response beyond human emotion.

While affect, by virtue of being a state of stimulation which is oftentimes so interwoven with our everyday existence that it becomes difficult to recognize or account for, is often discussed in terms of its outward bodily manifestations, this is not to say that it completely evades cognition. The two interact in subtle ways. Gregg and Seigworth (2010) clarify this point by noting that "sensate tendrils constantly extend between unconscious (or, better, non-conscious) affect and conscious thought" (2–3), thus, never fully separating them. Affect allows us to approach social phenomena, such as those described by Durkheim, in more nuanced ways by opening up new angles for understanding previously overlooked micro-encounters and unnoticed stimuli in combination with individual emotive responses and perceived meanings. Thus, the study of affect illustrates an avenue through which deeply personal and fundamentally social responses may be simultaneously articulated. In short, musicking stirs within us primordial affective experiences and emotions, creating connections with others and affirming social bonds, which in turn fuels further affective stimulation. The personal and the social necessitate one another to achieve the kinds of emotional responses that are so commonly associated with music.

Affect is fundamentally connected to our experience of life, the "messiness of the experiential" (Ahmed 2010, 571). Within an affective process, distinctions between external stimuli and internal responses quickly become blurred, particularly within those affective environments in which multiple bodies and environmental stimuli are connected in psycho-physiological reciprocity or co-participation. The bodily responses elicited through affective cues should be thought of as fundamentally connected to relations and encounters with the world, and given the importance placed by Small (1998) on person-to-person relationships and encounters, or those between people and wider society, any understanding of musically motivated person-to-person intensities should also consider their affective nature. Moreover, the terms that are typically used to describe our emotional states do not adequately describe the variety of affective responses, scenes, or events that humans may experience (Wetherell 2012).

This is not to say, however, that affect and emotions are not intimately linked. How we experience emotions can be a profoundly social phenomenon; they are felt through interpersonal interaction from some of our earliest stages of development during infancy. These emotionally profound interactions are often musical in nature, exhibiting characteristics of speech and movement generally not found elsewhere such as unusual rhythm or pulse, pitch, or elongated and exaggerated annunciation or duration. This phenomenon has been referred to as "communicative musicality" (Malloch 1999, 47). Such musicality is applied across the world, in various cultural contexts, and represents some of the most basic forms of embodied interpersonal communication between infants and caregivers (Krueger 2014). What this suggests is that empathic musical communication seems to be hardwired into our earliest development. There is something more universal about how we respond to musical stimuli than is often readily acknowledged and, further, it begins to shed light on how music is able to occupy the more emotional avenues of our minds, even when exposed to previously unheard music.

It is now possible to store and share tens of thousands of songs on our smartphones. What Small (1998) would refer to as the organized sound of musical meaning is now highly portable and may be flexibly introduced into a variety of settings through intuitive and easy-to-use technologies (DeNora 2013). And given that affective responses are likely to result from ill-defined or unnoticed cues, music—being an everyday phenomenon that is present in all cultures and walks of life—can be understood to be a potent medium through which Gregg and Seigworth's minuscule and molecular events of the unnoticed may be compounded into larger affective and collective responses such as the accounts of Australian rituals presented by Durkheim. In this regard, and given the deeply affective qualities of music, it would seem that affective musical experiences are able to contribute to the creation of effervescent assemblies through co-performance and musicking.

With all of this in mind, the theory of musical effervescence can now begin to take a more concrete shape. At the outset of this chapter, I noted that Durkheim's analysis of collective effervescence makes a number of references to songs, chants, rhythms, dances, and various other forms of cultural expression. While Durkheim dismisses the musical and rhythmic manifestations of the observed effervescent assemblies, it is, in my own opinion, a considerable oversight to ignore the profoundly effervescent and interpersonal nature of musicking that appears to be deeply rooted within our evolutionary journey into modern humans. Put simply, the musical elements of collective effervescence are not byproducts of some larger process at work, but rather both integral to understanding the socio-psychological elements of the phenomenon as well as demonstrative of the importance of musicking as an expression of our shared human experience.

Developing upon Durkheim's theory, musical effervescence can be thought of as a phenomenon that may occur when individuals come together and make music within the context of shared goals, beliefs, and/or needs. This impetus must be sufficiently powerful to mobilize a sense of purpose among the participants (consciously or otherwise). Through the sharing of these musical experiences, spatial and temporal connections between individuals engender both physical proximity between bodies as well as an immediacy to the aforementioned purpose. Synchronized bodies become entrained minds as the musical-empathic overlaps in the geographies of the brain encourage the sharing of emotions and ideals through verbal, nonverbal, and embodied cues. Affected states of being that are common in many musicking experiences are heightened by way of interconnectivity with others, leading to the sonorous, and physical signs of effervescence. Finally, with the body and mind in an energized state, Durkheim's manic creativity nourishes the formulation of new social relationships and ways of being in the world as viewed through the lens of the original purpose (see Figure 3.1). Broadly speaking, musical effervescence can be a powerful catalyst for change, harnessing some of our most ancient neurochemical pathways and socio-biological imperatives (to give voice to emotions and strengthen connections between members of a community through music) in order to cultivate transformative experiences that—in some cases—can gather the momentum needed to manifest into wider societal change.

The concept of musical effervescence is without question built upon the foundation of Durkheim's work, but it would be a superficial reading to consider the approach merely a footnote to his design. It is highly improbable that we will ever know if the collective effervescence observed by Durkheim was fueled, even in part, by song, dance, and procession by torchlight. But we can piece together a framework for understanding the emotionally and physiologically stimulating properties of music that are simultaneously profoundly transformative and fascinatingly innocuous. Preexisting theories that have been proposed to describe affective states of intersubjectivity among large groups of people—including collective effervescence (Durkheim [1912] 2008), interaction ritual chains (Collins 2004), or various crowd psychology theories (Le Bon [1895] 2009; Diener et al. 1980; Zimbardo 2008; Paulus 2015)—either consider their sonorous or musical qualities as byproducts of the intense interactions (as in the case of Durkheim) or

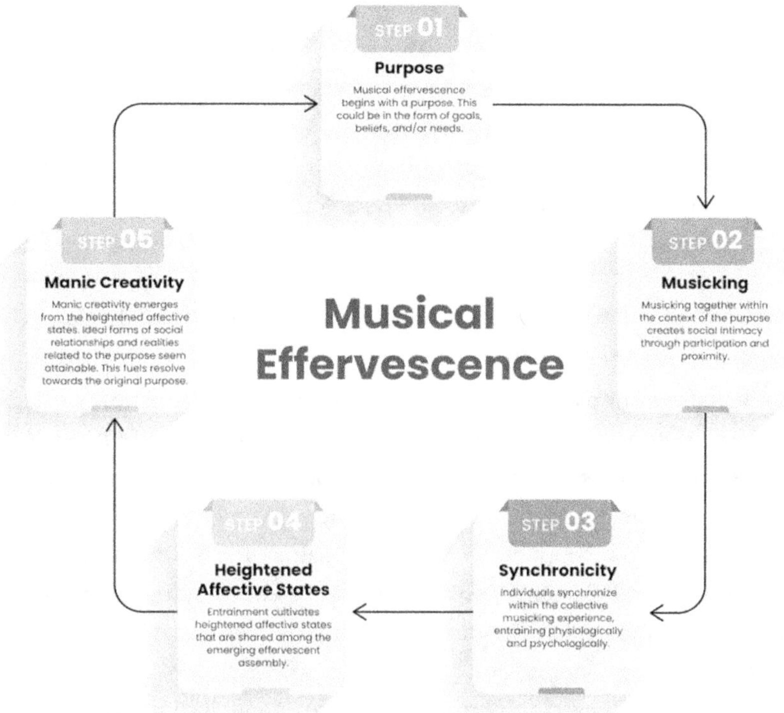

Figure 3.1 The process of musical effervescence. Image curated by the author.

do not meaningfully engage with them at all. While ethnomusicologists have—at times—flirted with the concept of effervescence to help explain their observations of some of the more animated musical rituals (see Seeger 1987), ethnomusicological theories, when considered alone, fall short of comprehensively accounting for the complex interplay of musical, psychological, physiological, and social factors that characterize musical effervescence (see Small 1998; Feld 1988; Keil and Feld 1994).

Within music performance, we find the building blocks of effervescence, and indeed, as Durkheim describes, within effervescent assemblies is the tendency toward embodied musical expression. As such, music can be thought of as both a facilitator and product of effervescence. Eons of human evolution have predisposed every one of us to tune in to the same micro-rhythms and emotive expressions of the human experience and synchronize within patterns of collective participatory performance. Such predispositions to synchronicity, emotive expressivity, vocal articulations, collective interaction, and participation provide the foundations for understanding some of the deeply personal, fundamentally social, and profoundly influential effects of music.

Musical effervescence capitalizes upon such predispositions and the psychological and physiological pathways that remain within us from the earliest days of musilanguage to cultivate an affectively charged heightened state of being. Manic creativity facilitates new possibilities of social relationships; social realities may be conceptualized and, as Turino noted, perceived to be not only attainable but also innate and true. Such realities, as discussed in this book, include those in which HIV medication is available to those who need it, where PLHIV need not live in fear of violence, and the burdens associated with the HIV/AIDS epidemic are lifted from the shoulders of South Africa's most vulnerable.

While these examples are of course consistent with the themes of this book, it would be a mistake to consider musical effervescence a uniquely African phenomenon or indeed that it is one that emerges exclusively within the domain of health emergencies and medical anthropology. As an analytical tool, musical effervescence may be applied to any participatory musicking event in which the aforementioned elements converge. Potential sites of musical effervescence are vast and may include Christian evangelical or gospel churches that employ music to uplift the congregation in animated worship, political rallies, protest movements, or various examples of participatory and spiritual trancing found across the world.

It has been my intention in this chapter to draw together this messy collection of conceptual threads into a coherent theory of musical effervescence for two purposes. The first has been to help account for the ways in which music can so easily animate us to embodied expression and heightened emotional states of being. The second has been in order to equip the reader with the knowledge to identify this same phenomenon, hiding in plain sight within a disparate array of performative responses to the South African AIDS crisis. It is with particular reference to this second purpose that the cultural importance of music across South Africa's diverse ethnic landscape—that is discussed in the following chapter—becomes an important prism through which to view such examples.

4

Song as Social Life and Cultural Armament

For as long as there has been scholarly writing about the African continent, there has been fascination with its musics. This chapter—while not an encyclopedic summary of South African musical history—has the unenviable task of distilling the complex interconnecting fabrics of long-established performance practices, settler colonialism, and music-making into a small handful of printed pages. I do this because this book presents a series of analyses of the songs that have been employed by South Africans within the HIV/AIDS epidemic, which benefit from a generalized understanding of South African cultural heritage. As such, the chapter serves as a platform from which one might better understand the cultural importance of song and singing in South Africa so that discussions of the various applications of song within the AIDS epidemic in later chapters are adequately contextualized. Without a strong grasp of why songs are such a fundamental component to South African cultural identity, the intricacies of their reappropriation in the struggle against HIV may be obscured.

This chapter will make numerous references to traditional music, but the concept of tradition in South Africa is complex and problematized by the politics of race and a history of subjugation. Through contact with European explorers and settlers, the erosion and/or manipulation of local cultural and musical life was a common experience among the many peoples who inhabited—willingly or otherwise—the land now known as South Africa. To paraphrase the noted South African musicologist Christopher Ballantine (1993), from the very beginning of European contact with the peoples of Southern Africa, the musics that have developed have been a fusion of styles that the colonial system thrust together.

Examples of this can be found in the earliest years of European settlement of the Cape, in which slaves from as far as Java, Madagascar, India, and elsewhere had their indigenous languages, customs, identities, and musics eroded as they were forcibly and administratively grouped together with the nomadic Khoikhoi and San peoples under the legal racial designation of Coloured (Coplan 1985).

The creole musical styles that appeared during this time have developed into traditional South African genres of their own in the form of *klopse* minstrelsy,[1] ghoema,[2] and Cape jazz,[3] among others (Martin 2013).

Under the apartheid system, the local customs of South Africa's Black cultures were both sites of identity and cultural pride for their peoples, while simultaneously heralded by the state as evidence of insurmountable ethnic and racial division entrenched by the regime (Kivnick 1990). These practices, however, also functioned as the bedrock from which agency, identity, and community bonds could be cultivated to push back against an antagonistic and belligerent state. One of the most striking problems facing those concerned with the study of tradition in South Africa, particularly in the colonial and apartheid eras, is that the tools of oppression and liberation were often fashioned from the same materials (Olsen 2014).

While these ambiguities render simplistic evaluations of traditional South African performance culture impossible, the cultural significance of songs, and the performing arts more generally, must be discussed before any exploration of their application within the context of HIV/AIDS. While books could be—and have been—written on this subject alone, it is still possible to briefly discuss the importance of music in South Africa's history, cultures, politics, and social life.

Songs in Social and Cultural Life

Various cultures across the African continent have been using performance, music, song, and dance to facilitate community education and develop social relationships for generations (Kivnick 1990). South Africa is no exception to this, and one feature that may be said to sit at the heart of much South African music is singing. While drumming is often associated with popular Western conceptions of a nebulous and undefined "African music," (Muller 2008)[4] singing is the dominant form of music-making in South Africa.[5] Songs, and the performing arts more generally, often play vital roles in social cohesion and cultural unity, preserving the social structures that hold communities together. They maintain important functions in many ceremonies, initiations, rites of passage, and rituals (Kivnick 1990; Blacking 1985; Erlmann 1991; Meintjes 2004; McNeill 2011). As Kivncik notes of the Venda and Tsonga-speaking peoples (but applicable to many of the country's cultures), "all men, women, and children participate in music making as part of involvement in other cultural activities" (1990: 94).

As has been noted by previous scholars of South African music (Kivnick 1990), members of a society, broadly speaking, learn the principles of their music and dance through the process of socialization. That is to say, as members learn to function within their society, they also learn, almost as a by-product of social maturation, the performance-based aspects of community life. Many examples of this can be found across South Africa. Music and dance are used in Xhosa female initiations known as *Ukuthombisa*, a performance ritual that prepares a young woman for adulthood and marriage (Sirayi 2012, 64). Each ritual is performed with elaborate costumes worn for the purpose of entertaining the audience, both humans and spirits (Sirayi 2012). South African drama theorist Mzo Sirayi notes that singing and dancing play important roles in the ritual for education and initiation, remarking that the songs involved in the process "are sung for joy and for sex education" (2012, 65). Importantly, these initiation songs bring together two main themes of this book: joy (or at least some form of strong emotional or affective connection to the message and subject matter of the initiation) and sexual health education. Implied within Sirayi's description of the purpose of the ritual is that the function of the songs (to educate initiates on aspects of womanhood, including reproductive health) is fundamentally connected to the emotional expressions of the music. The lyrics of these local songs contain knowledge to be passed on in prescribed ways, largely through interactive group performances. While initiates are kept in isolation for many days as part of the initiation, much of the ritual is performed to the community and thus the event bears many of the elements that educational campaign organizations strive for: entertainment, educational material, emotive or moving content, and group participation.

Further examples can be found within Zulu cultural activities. Ethnomusicologist Louise Meintjes (2004) notes that Zulu *ingoma* dance rituals, usually performed during social transition ceremonies such as initiations or weddings, are "integrally tied to an expression of Zulu-ness in song and dance" (177). The term *ingoma*—used in many Bantu languages across sub-Saharan Africa and not exclusive to the isiZulu language—covers a wide range of male performance music and group dances. Anthropologist Veit Erlmann (1991) suggests that the "patterns of *ingoma* are inseparably linked to choral songs in call and response structure, and as such constitute a complex statement of the unity of dance and song in Zulu performance culture" (95).

These dance songs developed from competitive group activities such as *iJadu*. The *iJadu* activities are an ancient tradition that served two main purposes within the Zulu communities. The first related to athleticism and play, providing a forum through which adolescents in the community could publicly display their physical prowess. The second purpose, and that with which *iJadu* is the most commonly associated, is as inter-clan match-making for those of marriageable age. As Bryant (1949) notes in an early and wide-ranging exploration of Zulu culture, exogamy was a common practice among precolonial Zulu communities, and suitable pretenses to bring different communities together had to be found. The young men and women of different clans would arrange to meet, ostensibly to compete with one another, but also with the purpose of becoming personally acquainted. These competitions played crucial roles in maintaining healthy social reproduction and strengthening bonds among clans.

When considering the importance of song within traditional South African cultures, the Venda rituals of the northern Limpopo province have also been the subject of a great deal of ethnomusicological and anthropological interest. Some of the most noteworthy of these include John Blacking's *Venda Children's Songs* (1967), Fraser McNeill's *AIDS, Politics, and Music in South Africa* (2011), and Helen Kivnick's *Where Is the Way?* (1990). The region was one of the last in South Africa to be influenced by European contact, with Blacking (1967) noting in the late 1960s that "the influence of Europeans remains relatively superficial" (16). This lack of contact with European colonists allowed for the relative preservation of local Venda cultural life well into the twentieth century, a time when other South African cultures had already endured the erosion associated with over a hundred years of colonial exploitation.

Within some cultural epistemologies, birth and death are cyclically connected, as each newborn baby is thought to represent the return of an ancestor. The rituals that surround this cycle support cultural understandings of life and death, with music permeating each of the activities that facilitate harmony in the community (Kivnick 1990). Of these, it is perhaps *Domba* that is the most famous of the Venda rituals due to the "Python Dance" in which male and female participants dance separately in fluid rows imitating snakelike movements. Throughout this rite, participants perform specific dances in symbolic formations while singing, often in elaborate polyphony, to vigorous and rhythmic drum accompaniment, while men are encouraged to scout for potential future wives in the female snake (Blacking 1985).

The *Domba* performance helps to facilitate control and maintenance of the social order within and between Venda communities. It bears significant symbolic meaning for social health insofar as it may be understood as figurative abstractions of the physical acts of sexual and social reproduction. Within *Domba*, the boundaries between participants and ancestral spirits are blurred, affording the ritual a spiritual as well as practical social purpose (Blacking 1969, 1985). McNeill warns not to consider this adoption of ancestral personae in abstract terms, noting, for instance, that various aspects of the ritual—including garments and decorative adornments—are thought to quite literally transform the girls into powerful manifestations of female ancestors. As a result, *Domba* presents a potent example of performance as a cultural imperative for the ongoing maintenance of the social fabric of the community. It further illustrates that separating South African artistic expression into Western pigeonholes risks stripping those performance practices of their cultural significance. In the case of *Domba*, the ritual could not be completed if one element (drumming, dancing, garments, songs, etc.) were to be removed.

Young women can only perform the songs and dances associated with specific rituals of ceremonial initiation into womanhood after their first menses (McNeill 2011). It is in such rituals that women are taught how to manage this newly acquired reproductive function. Thus, these rituals form pillars around which social life in many Venda communities is constructed, sex education is transferred, and life skills are taught to newly initiated adults. As McNeill notes, similarly to the Xhosa *Ukuthombisa* ritual discussed earlier in this chapter, the "boundaries between ancestral spirits and human beings are blurred in the interests of maximizing conditions for the promotion of fertility and the reproduction of 'the Venda nation'" (76). By blurring such boundaries of reality, information considered taboo, dangerous, or powerful, such as knowledge concerning reproduction and fertility, might be safely transferred from one generation to the next.

Importantly for any discussion around HIV/AIDS, these rites form part of the education on ritual knowledge of womanhood, managing the issues that will influence their lives in their new societal roles as adult members of their community. Ancestral knowledge, and the authority to wield such knowledge, plays key roles in health education for those who are coming of age. With specific reference to AIDS, epidemic prevention in such communities is predicated less on biomedical knowledge than on the abilities of gifted divinators and bearers of ancestral knowledge—usually community elders—to apply their wisdom (McNeill 2011).

Many of the songs that have permeated across South African social life are structured in call-and-response patterns, what is known in the Western classical canon as antecedent and consequent. Such patterns reflect the nature of the songs as social acts, as they are inclusive and conducive to participation. They often are reflective of the minutiae of everyday life and act as outlets for the kinds of human emotions and experiences that can be found in communities all over the world. The choruses may reflect issues of joy or celebration—as in the case of weddings or childbirth—or loss and sorrow—as in the case of funerals or the loss of one's ancestral lands. While the direct and indirect influence of the migrant labor system noted in Chapter 2 on South African music will be discussed later, it should be mentioned here that the songs also gave voice to expressions of support and solidarity among women who were often left alone while the men worked in the cities, particularly during the peak of these labor migrations under the apartheid system.

South Africa's oral knowledge has been, and continues to be, transmitted from person to person and committed to memory for future generations to learn. The significance of these oral narratives cannot be overstated, since they are often the main vehicle for the continuation of information and wisdom accumulated over generations. A particularly powerful quote from Tshifiwe, a learned and respected Venda culture bearer in spite of his humble occupation as a janitor at the then State University of the Republic of Venda, that appears in Kivnick's work highlights this fact.

> These songs really tell you something. Even if it's kids playing, you find it has a meaning in it. And when those kids are playing and singing their own songs, they are practicing, so to say, for the music of our people. Even when they are just playing, their songs are teaching them to be Vendas. (Kivnick 1990, 83)

Tshifiwe's words demonstrate the important connections between songs and cultural identity, and while speaking in relation to the Venda people, similar views can be found across South Africa's many cultures.

Christianity and Church Songs

The vast majority of South Africans self-identify as Christian, with many of the denominations of Christianity in the country blending with local belief systems to form syncretic faiths. As such, it is difficult to discuss music-making in South Africa, and singing in particular, without discussing (albeit briefly) the Christian missions that carved out spaces across the land. Exerting enormous influence on the performance cultures of the local peoples over the centuries, stylistic, thematic, and performative aspects of Christian worship can be found throughout South Africa's vast repertoires of traditional music.

While the first missionaries began proselytizing in the Cape in the seventeenth century, it was not until the nineteenth century that missions were established deep into the heartlands of the region (Oosthuizen 1968). The goal of the missions across the frontiers of Southern Africa, while not uniform in their approach, has been generally understood as a so-called civilizing pursuit to spread the Christian faith, and one that wrought destruction on the local epistemologies and cultures of the various peoples that inhabited the land prior to settlement (Chikowero 2015). Within this context of European settler colonialism, the introduction of Christianity threatened the social fabric of local communities, and the rapid development of Christian communities represented a growing challenge both to ancestral knowledge and claims to authority by village chiefs.

In order to be considered Christian, South Africans had to join a mission church. This often meant that newly converted Christians were separated from their former community to limit the possibility of being influenced by their former customs and ways of life (Dargie 1997). Initially drawing their congregation from social outcasts, those accused of witchcraft or other evils, and the abandoned, the popularity of the new religion quickly began to attract members from beyond this pool of individuals. As the mission biographer John A. Chalmers (1878) noted in the late nineteenth century, by physically separating the congregants from their former homes, the missionaries filled the positions of moral and political authority and began to rival the power of the local chiefs.

Noting the prevalence of community singing among the local populations, these early religious leaders quickly wrapped their message of Christianity in music. Not the music made by the local communities, which was often viewed with suspicion and derision by the missionaries, but rather in the form of Wesleyan hymns. Their goal was often to replace previous forms of music-making within the communities with morally and religiously acceptable alternatives—which, of course, would be the vessels for their specific approach to the divine. While the missions were in many ways successful in erasing much of the local ways of being across Southern Africa (Chikowero 2015), a number of communities began to incorporate elements of their own musical cultures within the hymns.

Of the early converts to Christianity, Ntsikana Gaba, an isiXhosa-speaking composer and poet, is perhaps one of the most well-known for his influence on the development of a distinctly South African form of Christianity and style of hymn singing (Muller 2008). Persuaded to displace some aspects of Xhosa culture and replace them with Christian teachings, his approach is one of the earliest representations of syncretism among South Africa's Christian communities. This syncretism can be heard within the music he composed that has been passed down through generations of isiXhosa-speaking Christians. These hymns adopted many of the characteristics of precolonial Xhosa songs such as parallel movement among vocal lines and the use of clapping or other rhythmic devices.

Syncretic faiths, often with a prophet at the head of the church, quickly became a model that was appropriated by different groups across the newly developing country, with notable examples including The Ethiopians, The Nazareth Baptist Church, and various faith groups that splintered from the Christian Catholic Apostolic Church in Zion. The idea of a messianic figure who, despite his abuse and eventual death at the hands of the authorities, rose to triumph was deeply appealing to communities increasingly under pressure from colonial administrations. Moreover, anger at the prevailing belief among mission teachings that Africa had no history or culture of value prior to European colonization prompted a gradual shift away from the mission ideology.

With the introduction of Bibles translated into local languages, the development of Africanized expressions of faith became more commonplace. Melodies would be borrowed from familiar folk tunes, with singers employing call-and-response patterns, often continuing the melody to overlap with the following musical phrase. Improvisation was encouraged from the lead vocalist voicing the antecedent, and the cyclical nature of the patterns afforded the freedom for exploring individualized expressions of faith and increased communal participation.

Dance also emerged as an important element of South African Christian demonstrations of worship (Muller 2008). In the early twentieth century, the charismatic leader of the Nazarites, Isaiah Shembe, created a new style of sacred singing and dancing, one that was rooted in both local culture and beliefs and Christian spirituality. This was characteristic of Shembe's approach to spiritual life and worship, one that was inspired by the pioneering approach to expressions of Christian faith of Ntsikana Gaba and stood in stark opposition to the quest to civilize and Westernize South African communities that was promoted by the majority of missions. In addition to introducing cultural pillars of local South African life, such as the veneration of ancestors, Shembe further distanced his church from those of the Europeans by introducing performance into expressions of worship in the form of *umgidi*, the sacred dance (Sithole 2014). This was particularly out of the ordinary for the time, as religious dance rituals had been discouraged as uncivilized and unchristian by the missionaries (Muller 2008).

The dance involved many aural and visual hallmarks of precolonial rituals, including choreography, costume, and singing. These newly composed poetic forms made explicit reference to the experiences of Black South Africans under White minority rule, blurring the boundaries between religious, social, and political life. Indeed, much of the political frustrations of the time were channeled into the independent Christian movements that had split from the teachings of the European missions, as these politically minded faith groups were more readily tolerated by colonial—and later apartheid—governments than would be the case for a secular political movement (Oosthuisen 1968).

Another influential Christian movement adopted the moniker of The Ethiopians, as a result of the numerous references to Ethiopia in the Bible. While the history of this spiritual movement is difficult to precisely determine, the 1892 resignation of Black South African minister Mangena Mokone from the Wesleyan Church is considered as a turning point in the story (Muller 2008). Establishing his own church, which he named The Ethiopians, his departure sparked a series of protest resignations across the Cape missions in response to racial discrimination. Mokone developed strong ties with American churches and demonstrated that the European domination of Christianity in Southern Africa could be challenged. By the early nineteenth century, the Xhosa prophet Ntsikana Gaba mentioned earlier in this chapter had become associated with The Ethiopians, strengthening the movement's reputation and practices as an African church. Indeed, as Muller (2008) explains, strong connections were formed between these churches and the development of a Black South African political consciousness.

> Many Ethiopianists joined together in 1909 to form the Ntsikana Memorial Association, a cultural, rather than religious, organization that constituted a starting point for the formation of what later became the African National Congress. Out of this movement came the Enoch Sontonga composition, "Nkosi Sikelel'iAfrika" ("God Bless Africa"), adopted as the anthem of the African

> National Congress in 1925 and now a central part of the South African national anthem. (96–7)

Developed in a social and political climate of racial intolerance, settler colonialism, and radical social engineering, this example highlights that the boundaries between religious, political, and folk songs are often nebulous and permeable, as will be noted in more detail later in this chapter.

By drawing culturally and stylistically from local customs and mission teachings, the religious expressions that have emerged from South Africa's syncretic faiths represent a powerful manifestation of local cultural identity within the structures of state-sponsored cultural erasure. Moreover, churches would become centers around which communities, interconnected through their shared faith and local bonds, could organize in opposition to increasingly repressive White minority governments. By blending local epistemologies and ways of being with Christian beliefs, the congregations typically exhibited many of the signs associated with musical effervescence discussed in Chapter 3. Indeed, it is no coincidence that communal singing is often associated with some of the most exuberant displays of faith and worship. Focused attention, group participation, and the introduction of local cultural rhythmic elements provide important foundations from which effervescence may be cultivated and then harnessed for political mobilization. The church became a space in which Black South Africans could reclaim a sense of personhood and purpose through faith and song. It became a cleansing force within an environment that sought to taint Other Black individuals. As scholars have noted, the physical liberation of the burden of oppression was achieved not just through worship and prayer, but through communal song and dance (Kivnick 1990).

Songs and the Migrant Labor System

While songs characterize the narrative of community life, so too do they characterize the lives of the men who must leave their homes. Toward the end of the nineteenth century, the mining industry in South Africa grew at a tremendous rate, creating a demand for labor that drew migrants from across sub-Saharan Africa. As noted in Chapter 2, South Africa's wealth was built upon the exploitation of human capital. The foundation of this exploitation lay within the migrant labor system that saw thousands of men leave their rural homes to work in the various gold mines around the city of Johannesburg. The imposition of colonial taxation, coupled with few economic opportunities for Black South Africans, left few other options to make a living. It was those communities most affected by the aforementioned Christian missions who were the most vulnerable to such exploitation, and subsequently, vast collections of migrant workers with different values, customs, languages, levels of education, world views, social orders, epistemologies, beliefs, and ways of being found themselves thrust together in shared hostel accommodation (Coplan 1985).

One of the results of this melting pot of cultures was the development of a diverse repertoire of performance cultures. Due to the lengthy, yet inconsistent contracts, continuous movement between rural homes and urban work ensured the flow of new cultural input. While still drawing inspiration from their cultural roots, new identities were formed that forewent ethnic divisions and instead focused on their developing urban identities. As Coplan (1985) notes, as new musical expressions evolved in rural South Africa in response to the emerging realities, the performance spaces in the areas around the mines also "became the crucibles of creativity and dissemination" (407).

While certainly not the only form of music to develop as a result of the migrant labor system, the Zulu male vocal style known as *isicathamiya*—popularized globally by the internationally acclaimed Ladysmith Black Mambazo in the 1980s—is perhaps one of the most well-known examples. This genre of Zulu choral singing has been explored in great detail by scholars of South Africa's performance culture, including in Veit Erlmann's *Nightsong* (1991) and David Coplan's *In Township Tonight* (1985). It is not my intention to repackage what is already well-trodden ground within South African performance and cultural studies, but it is nevertheless important to provide points of contact that demonstrate how various performing arts—with particular focus on singing—have emerged from specific social and economic circumstances to take on important roles in social life and cultural armament, that is to say the use of culture in collective self-defense. This particular section highlights the development of art forms that reflected the restructuring of South Africa's precapitalist forms of social organization under colonial rule and the influence of heterogeneous cultural resources that resulted from migrancy.

The history and development of *isicathamiya*, as with many of South Africa's traditional musics, remains contested but is generally considered to have its roots in the *iJadu* dance singing competitions discussed earlier in this chapter and the Zulu choral styles of *mbube*—popularized by vocal group Solomon Linda and the Original Evening Birds—and later *ingoma busuku* (Erlmann 1991). A key difference between the styles can be found in their performance practices, while *mbube* singers strive for powerful vocal performances, *isicathamiya* performers are generally more concerned with intricate harmonious call-and-response patterns between the lead falsetto singer and his accompaniment.

Typically, *isicathamiya* is characterized by its close a cappella harmonies and carefully choreographed dance routines inspired by traditional Zulu dances. These elegant movements would prioritize smaller and more gentle movements than their traditional counterparts, resulting in the name *isicathamiya*, which translates roughly to mean "tiptoe guys" (Erlmann 1996). The exclusively male-voice choirs blended precolonial polyphonic part-singing with choral music introduced by Christian missions. Their lyrics often dealt with the harsh realities of life in the mines and included topics such as working conditions, inter-clan conflicts, religious faith, social problems introduced by the migrant labor system, and the indignities wrought by White minority rule (Erlmann 1996). As South African choral music scholar Mollie Stone (2015) notes, singing *isicathamiya* helped workers communalize the psychological and emotional burdens of their lives. This propensity of participatory musicking to connect individuals together and collectivize trauma will become important to the discussions of how PLHIV used music to cope with the burdens of AIDS in later chapters. Moreover, much like their counterparts during the liberation struggle, many of the songs served to venerate specific individuals or groups. In this case, it was those who labored in the mines who were praised for their strength and courage. This practice can be attributed not simply to previous forms of singing but also to earlier traditions of praise poetry, which saw orators recite family lineages, provide reverence to ancestors, or praise the achievements of highly accomplished individuals (Stone 2015).

Isicathamiya emerged at a time of increasing urbanization of rural Black South Africans and exposure to African American performance culture. American minstrel shows had become extremely popular throughout South Africa, particularly in the rapidly expanding urban centers, with Orpheus McAdoo's Virginia Jubilee Singers and later the Minstrel, Vaudeville and Concert Company becoming household names (Erlmann 1990). During the twentieth century, according to Ballantine (1993), "for several decades, urban South Africans were held in thrall by American culture—but above all by the activities and achievements of blacks in that society. Where American culture fascinated, *black* American culture infatuated" (13). This fascination with

African American culture would bring with it some of the sounds that would become synonymous with social and political mobilization such as jazz and later soul. These sounds would go on to become associated with the expressive content of the budding American Civil Rights Movement, obscuring the boundaries between music for entertainment, religion, and politics (Muller 2008).

McAdoo's performances and others like them could be heard in the migrant compounds around South Africa's mines, where the audiences would comprise miners, laborers, and other migrant workers. *Isicathamiya* blended stylistic qualities from rural dance singing competitions, American vaudeville, and ragtime, to create a sound that represented and reflected the circulating rural-to-urban movement—and the subsequent blurring of those spheres of life—that characterized South Africa's political economy.

With the loss of ancestral lands and the harsh realities of migrant life, *isicathamiya* performances in migrant communities provided more than simply a means through which to mourn the loss of their lands and dignity. Instead, the performers drew from their respective cultural backgrounds to create stylistic vehicles through which to bring structure and meaning to a world of systematic oppression and indifference to human suffering. These performance spaces became environments through which emotional resilience and resistance could be cultivated.

Fast forward to nearly a century later, and these same traditional songs have been applied within South Africa's AIDS crisis as a means of suspending hierarchical social orders so that younger voices may be heard. As anthropologist Liz Gunner (2003) notes, the popularity of the *isicathamiya* genre has been harnessed by young men to address HIV/AIDS-related issues that would not normally be permissible outside the specific nexus of song.

> The gravitas which the genre can command means that even very young groups who enter into its performance space, its specific modality, become invested with its authority. Thus a group of extremely youthful singers can sing with the same fervour as older groups, yet bring to it a particular set of performance skills and command the attention of their audience. (42)

By expressing themselves through songs closely connected with Zulu traditional and historical identity, younger generations may draw legitimacy from the cultural authority associated with the genre. In doing so, they present their ideas within the framework of Zuluness. Not only are they able to address community members of much higher social status but also present information on issues that may otherwise be considered restricted or taboo subjects.

Isicathamiya is only one example of a music that developed as a result of the migrant labor system, but it presents an important illustration of how Black South Africans reclaimed agency and cultural identity through song. The environments cultivated by these a cappella competitions invoked a cultural heritage of Zuluness that spanned generations as well as the influence of a burgeoning American Civil Rights Movement to create a socio-sonic bricolage of semiotic affordances that would contribute to the development of some of South Africa's most iconic music, the songs of the liberation struggle.

Songs and the Anti-Apartheid Struggle

The twentieth-century history of South Africa is undoubtedly dominated by the struggle against European colonization and apartheid. This period saw songs deployed as cultural weaponry and armor, as expressions of both collective suffering and faith, and reflect and sculpt the social and political landscape in ways that would eventually culminate in South Africa's first fully democratic elections. This may sound like hyperbole, and to be sure, the suggestion that songs alone brought the country's reign of White minority rule to an end would be a gross oversimplification of the social, economic, and political determinants that converged to free the nation from subjugation. But I stand by my assertion. Without songs—and the weight of their shared historical and cultural significance—it is almost inconceivable that South Africa's history would remain unaltered from the one we know today.

When discussing South Africa's repertoire of struggle songs, it can be difficult to pin down exactly what a struggle song is. Indeed, some definitions that can be found in the academic literature can be less than helpful. For example, one scholar has characterized them as "the ubiquitous but largely informal and un-professionalized genre that was probably the dominant musical medium of popular political expression" (Gilbert 2007, 423). Definitions such as these are of little analytical use, but they do provide an entry point for discussion.

Perhaps a more detailed account of struggle songs in South Africa would highlight that, while of course, they are songs the purpose of which is to vocalize (explicitly or otherwise) political or social commentary, they draw influence from across South Africa's musical landscape as a result of the blurred boundaries between traditional South African musical styles, church songs, and hymns—themselves often stylistic bricolages of African and European elements. Despite examples from the struggle repertoire that have individual composers, many songs are developed within local communities, often through numerous rounds of collective singing—in homes, small gatherings, or even in the moment at protests—in which ideas for themes or lyrics are piloted. Common practices include call-and-response patterns, thematic repetition, and multipart singing.

By the 1930s, the aforementioned influence of the American traveling vaudeville shows was giving way to more local musical forms that were being applied in overtly political ways. As Ballantine (1991) notes, this shift in creative output sought "to assert the belief that there was intrinsically a value in the adoption or incorporation of musical materials that were African" (145). The Second World War, as a period of high inflation and an increasing low-income urban population, propelled what were previously quiet murmurings of discontent into more confrontational attitudes that manifested in the form of boycotts and protests. This seed of New Africanism, an intellectual movement that promoted African identity, would eventually develop into the struggle for independence.

By the mid-1950s, the forced removals of Black and Coloured South Africans by the recently formed apartheid government (noted earlier in Chapter 2) were being implemented with increasing vigor across the country. Perhaps the most infamous of the removals involved the destruction of Sophiatown, a bustling multiracial suburb north of Johannesburg. With a reputation for its vibrant cultural life (Switzer 1997; Impey 2008), Sophiatown represented something that the administrators of the apartheid state could not ignore: the dynamism and eclecticism that emerged from a desegregated suburb so close to the beating heart of their perceived White nation. While plagued with many social issues such as crime and housing shortages, contemporary accounts of the suburb tell of a lively hub of artistic activity and of musical and literary expression.

Sophiatown not only revealed that South Africans of different races could coexist, but the cultural melting pot demonstrated the kind of vitality that could develop if communities were allowed to mix. With the forced removal of Sophiatown's residents to the Meadowlands suburb of Soweto, a township to the South-West of Johannesburg (the name So-we-to referencing its identity as the South-West township of Johannesburg), this cultural hub was destroyed. Suitable performance venues in these new townships were almost nonexistent, and the authorities that governed the arts and culture ensured musical and artistic outputs remained segregated. Moreover, the period saw the introduction of ethnically based radio stations that broadcasted their musical biases toward neo-traditional and religious music thought to represent the various—and importantly, separate—ethnicities of South Africa (Ballantine 1993).

While Sophiatown may have been bulldozed to the ground, its memory lives on in the art and culture that was developed there. One powerful example of this comes in the form of a protest song written by Strike Vilakazi entitled "Meadowlands." Sung in *tsotsitaal*—a vernacular derived from mixing words and phrases from various South African languages and spoken in the South African townships—the English translation presented to the authorities is as follows.

> Let's go, let's go, let's go to Meadowlands
> We'll work night and day, going straight to Meadowlands

With its upbeat jive rhythm, the song presents itself as an anthem supportive of the relocations, fooling members of the government into promoting the song and rewarding Vilakazi with housing approval (Ansell 2005). However, the government officials failed to understand the nuances of *tsotsitaal* that indicated to those familiar with the vernacular that the lyrics were being sung ironically. The residents of Sophiatown understood that the song represented a demonstration of resistance, highlighting the manner in which the arts can be utilized as tools of hidden resistance that will be discussed in more detail later in this chapter.

This period also witnessed the National Party government, with its vision of a grand apartheid, implement political and cultural repression on an unprecedented scale. Political organizations such as the African National Congress (ANC) and the Pan African Congress (PAC) were banned, and sixty-nine people were killed while protesting against the increasingly restrictive system of passing laws in 1960 that became known as the Sharpeville massacre. In the wake of this tragedy, a faction of the ANC developed into the paramilitary group *uMkhonto we Sizwe* (MK) or Spear of the Nation. The cultural outputs around this time began to reflect this shift toward militantism with the introduction of new material into the older liberation songs. As one MK activist notes in the documentary film *Amandla! A Revolution in Four-Part Harmony*, "the songs started, like, to begin to take on those overtones, just changing a word here, changing a word there. Putting an A.K. [47 assault rifle] there, taking out a bible there" (cited in Hirsch 2002).

Some of the most notable examples of figuratively swapping bibles for AKs in that period include the newly composed struggle song "Sobashiy'abazali", translated from isiZulu to mean "we will leave our parents." This song references the youth of South Africa leaving their parents to join the guerrilla training camps that MK set up in sympathetic neighboring countries. But perhaps the most iconic cultural manifestation that emerged at this time was toyi-toyi. In terms of embodied action, one can hardly find a better example than this Southern African dance chant. The dance is thought to have "originated on the guerrilla training grounds of Zimbabwe to keep up the endurance and the spirits of the freedom fighters" (Michie and Gamede 2013, 262), but emerged as a powerful and popular means of embodying the percussive intensity of many of the demonstrations against the apartheid state. Indeed, as Durkheim ([1912] 2008) has noted, both mournful and celebratory events share a number of traits conducive to emotional surges noted in collective effervescence.

> If mourning differs from the other forms of the positive cult, there is one feature in which it resembles them: it, too, is made up out of collective ceremonies which produce a state of collective effervescence among those who take part in them. The sentiments that are aroused are different, but the arousal is the same. (399)

It is therefore unsurprising that the vast struggle repertoire has been applied in service of performative expressions of a diverse range of emotions.

Toyi-toyi involves jogging, usually with knees relatively high, with the arms raised above the head while chanting rhythmically to a consistent pulse provided by the pace of the jog. The rhythms within the call-and-response structure are said to imitate the sound of gunfire, and the chants often praise noted veterans of the liberation struggle (Hirsch 2002). Jazz icon Hugh Masekela recalls that toyi-toyi was used as a way of intimidating the enemy: "Because we can't beat these people physically, you can scare the shit out of them with a song" (Hirsch 2002).

Toyi-toyi presents an overt example through which rhythm, pulse, and entrainment have engendered collective action. The dance and chants help to create connections between individuals and synchronize their movements. These connections arguably contributed to heightened emotional states and a sense of safety as a collective whole. As one liberation struggle activist recalls: "toyi-toyi made us not see the bullets and the guns that the whites used to shoot us" (cited in Michie and Gamede 2013, 262).

Throughout these shifts in political rhetoric, the performing arts—and songs in particular—both shaped and reflected the aspirations, feelings, and experiences of Black South Africans. Given the nature of the apartheid state's brutal response to dissent, the informality of this genre noted by Gilbert (2007) in her definition at the beginning of this section is unsurprising. In his book on the arts and political resistance, David Scott (1990) notes that songs and other oral traditions, "due simply to their means of transmission, offer a kind of seclusion, control, and even anonymity that make them ideal vehicles for cultural resistance" (160). Thus, collective singing can be thought of as a fluid and expressive tool through which counter ideologies and morale-boosting ideas or messages may be transmitted and impressed in the public consciousness while simultaneously evading standard methods of censorship that suppressed much of the country's recorded music. This was particularly important throughout the 1970s and 1980s as increasing government intrusion into political speech characterized the post-1976 era in the wake of the Soweto uprisings noted in Chapter 1.

While the government censors explicitly banned very few records, the sophisticated cooperation between various arms of the state apparatus, including the police and state-run radio stations (through which independent stations were intimidated into boycotting certain artists), effectively silenced those musicians whose music was considered a threat to the governing moral and political ideology. One prominent example of this can be found in the music of Roger Lucey. As a result of his political rhetoric, Lucey became the subject of intimidation and sabotage that involved frequent police raids on his home, interrogations, surveillance of his movements, and ensuring invitations to perform did not reach him (Drewett 2007).

This approach of threats and intimidation allowed the state some degree of plausible deniability toward the general public and international community on their record of freedom of artistic expression while simultaneously rendering silent any material deemed unpalatable to the regime. That is not to say, however, that songs that expressed dissent were not composed and performed. Despite the efforts of the state, many independent radio stations continued to operate, some from outside the borders of South Africa. Moreover, given that the censors largely—albeit not exclusively—scrutinized song lyrics for ideological compliance, creative dissent was driven into the realm of subtextual and obfuscated meaning.

When discussing the coded messages that can be presented through music and the arts, Scott (1990) suggests that in order to fully understand what he refers to as "hidden transcripts," that is, particular ways of speaking or behaving that appear deferent or compliant while simultaneously and covertly express discontent, it is important to understand the broader culture of the subordinate people. Strike Vilakazi's "Meadowlands," noted earlier in this section, is a powerful example of a hidden transcript. Much of the political action of subordinate groups requires some form of interpretation or community-level shared understanding of meaning as a result of the structures of power that prevent open expressions of discontent (Scott 1990). These expressions are intentionally designed to be cryptic for the purpose of plausible deniability. This requires experimentation and comes with considerable risk since one must rely on the ambiguities of language, interpretations of silence or non-silence in interactions or performances. The performing arts, and music in particular, became important vehicles for both overtly and covertly voicing dissent, as well as mobilizing large numbers of people toward political objectives during minority rule in South Africa.

Throughout the political struggle, songs were used to bring unity, strength, and purpose to those who felt they had none. South Africa's political activists would sing their liberation songs while in prison, facing the police, during trials, or just in everyday life in order to keep their morale high (Schumann 2008). The call-and-response structure of many of these songs, which has its roots in the precolonial singing and dancing noted earlier in the chapter and subsequently shaped by contact with European settlers, lends itself to participation (Bozzoli 2004). Participation allows for collective emotion and grieving. The practice reinforces a sense of community, as it did for generations among the nation's precolonial ancestors. This sense of interconnectedness, community, and connection to cultural roots helped to cultivate resilience in the face of an oppressive state.

When conventional channels of communication disappeared, songs took their place as the voice of the people. For Gilbert (2005), songs are "often created and disseminated orally, are easily remembered, and if popular can spread with remarkable rapidity across wide-ranging social and geographical landscapes" (11). In particular, songs could address specific issues, whether a specific politician, as in the case of "Naants' indod' emnyama, Verwoerd" ("Beware, Verwoerd"),[6] originally composed by MK activist and singer Vuyisile Mini, or the training of South African freedom fighters in neighboring countries, as in the case of "Shona Malanga" ("Shorten the Day"). In these two examples, the latter expresses far more of what Scott (1990) would refer to as a hidden transcript than the former, insofar as the meanings of "Shona Malanga" are obfuscated and encoded within the narratives of the song. "Shona Malanga" does not overtly reference the liberation struggle; it is a song popularized by domestic workers and the content describes their one day off per week, what they referred to as "Sheila's day" (Schumann 2008). But as struggle veteran Sifiso Ntuli notes, "the song was adapted to the condition we found ourselves in, so instead of saying: 'we'll meet on Thursday, on Sheila's day, it became, we'll meet where we would rather not meet, in the bushes with our bazookas'" (cited in Hirsch 2002). In this respect, Sheila's day became synonymous with coming together in solidarity and resistance to the state.

Many forms of South African music present layers of different meanings. The semi-improvisational, mosaic structure of traditional, religious, and popular songs (though I have already noted that the boundaries between these genres are often nebulous and overlapping) and their lyrics help to infer deeper levels of meaning (Allen 2003). Lyrics, however, are only one aspect of a song that can be interpreted as meaningful. Coded messages can be implanted within the sonorous qualities of music and reinforced through association with a particular group or cause.

Perhaps the most well-known example of this is the now-current South African national anthem "Nkosi sikelel' iAfrica." Penned in 1897 by composer and Methodist mission clergyman Enoch Sontonga, the hymn makes no lyrical reference to the country's political struggles. Regardless, it was still banned by the apartheid state due to its association with the ANC, as it was used to open and close their meetings. Thus, while lyrics can be profoundly important in commenting on social issues (Scott 1990), the significance of songs lies not only in their words. Meaning can be found embedded in melodic, rhythmic, and other sonorous qualities, which may also signify localized meanings, and provide the impetus for embodied action and forms of effervescence.

While distinguished pianist and composer Abdullah Ibrahim (previously known as Dollar Brand) notes in the documentary film *Amandla! A Revolution in Four-Part Harmony* (2002), that it is unlikely that there has ever been a liberation or protest movement that has not, at some stage, used music or song to rally people to their cause, keep up morale, or mourn those who have fallen or been arrested, South Africa's struggle repertoire presents a unique and complex tapestry of interwoven threads that run deep within the nation's cultural history and collective consciousness. The history of songs and struggle has become so integral to South African identity that it is impossible to separate the culture of the liberation struggle from the country's wider cultural identities.

Conclusion

The purpose of this chapter has been to illustrate the importance of songs across the spectrum of South African cultures. There is a long history of applying the performing arts to effect social and political change, educate community members on specific issues, and build community cohesion that both long predates the written records of colonial settlers and stretches into the present day. When considering the use of songs and the performing arts as vehicles to communicate on the subject of HIV/AIDS throughout the years of the epidemic, it is important to recognize that similar practices have been applied to health communication, community mobilization, and collective psychosocial healing and grief processing for generations. It is within this rich history of music-related and music-driven social and political change that this book analyzes the mechanics of sonically embodied action within South Africa's AIDS crisis.

Symbolism and the propensity for songs to soak up meanings and associations and retain them as they are passed from generation to generation provide a powerful vehicle through which to develop health awareness and prevention strategies. Once symbolism has been established, the original symbol need not be present, or even exist, for the invocation of such symbols to generate the kinds of emotional energy discussed in Chapter 3. Thus, the cultural history of songs in South Africa provides fertile soil for forms of embodied action fueled by generations of local, community, and national participation in musical performance.

I have broadly highlighted the cultural importance of music in South Africa as a way to contextualize the use of such methods for health and social outcomes. But the application of music as a form of public health intervention within the country's AIDS epidemic does not occur in a geopolitical vacuum. Established forms of Western biomedical health and social messaging have interacted with local music-making traditions, informing the ways in which communities, organizations, and individuals perform and interpret these musically driven interventions. In order to understand the ways in which certain approaches are employed within the AIDS crisis—and the rationale for using them—it is useful to acknowledge how and why such approaches became popular means of public health promotion.

Notes

1 Kaapse Klopse (literally translated from Afrikaans to mean Cape Club) is the name given to groups of musicians who perform in the Cape Town Minstrel Carnival. The festival is held every year on January 2nd. Influenced by the American minstrels that visited South Africa in the late nineteenth and early twentieth centuries, colonial marching bands, and musical customs imported through the Indian Ocean slave routes, Klopse music traces its origin to New Year celebrations among Cape Town's slaves as they were only given time off to celebrate on January 2nd (Gaulier and Martin 2017). As a result, it is known informally as Tweede Nuwe Jaar (Second New Year).

2 Ghoema refers to a particular rhythm characterized by syncopation and played on a two-headed barrel drum that is strongly associated with klopse music (for more information, see Bruinders 2010 and Martin 2013).

3 Influenced by American jazz, Cape jazz is a style of music that emerged in the twentieth century under a political climate of repression, and built upon the creole culture that developed in the Cape Colony that is noted in Chapter 2 (Martin 2013).

4 Typically, this is influenced by the explosion of the world music industry in the 1980s, the popularity of West African artists and styles within that industry, the prevalence of drums across West African musical styles, and a generalized Western ignorance of the various musics of the African continent.

5 It is important to note here that while drumming does exist within the cultural repertoires of Southern Africa such as in Venda initiation rites (Blacking, Byron, and Nettl 1995) or the aforementioned klopse ghoema, its use is not as common as in other regions of Africa.

6 "Naants' indod'emnyama, Verwoerd" makes specific reference to Hendrik Verwoerd, a South African politician who served as Prime Minister of, first, The Union of South Africa (1958–61), and later The Republic of South Africa (1961–6) before being assassinated while in office. He is considered the "architect of apartheid" for his major role in the implementation of the country's apartheid system (Waldmeir 1998, 253).

5

Edutainment, Celebrity Advocacy, and the Legacy of Live Aid

The late morning sun streams into the office through a length of paned windows, casting crisscrossed shadows over the walls as velvety red curtains dance in the breeze from an open window. The room is decorated with various Southern African ornaments, and a large patterned rug leads toward two luxurious armchairs with intricately embroidered padding. The ambience is open and welcoming. I can feel the warmth of the Western Cape sunshine on my face and it reflects off the many glass photo frames that dress the office walls. In each of them is the same person, smiling broadly and genuinely, and often with company: Professor Jimmie Earl Perry, Director of Educational Theatre and Creative Arts at The ACHAM, Stellenbosch University. As I sit on one of the armchairs on the other side of a dark hardwood desk, I listen carefully to his considered thoughts on communicating through the performing arts.

> What we have done, certainly not on as large a scale as 46664, is present a mass awareness event that tries to do a similar thing: basically, make people aware that the virus still exists and you have a responsibility to help it go away, that's the bottom line.

He pauses for a second, as if choosing his words wisely, and momentarily glances at the phone sitting on the desk between us, innocuously recording every flutter of the curtains, shuffle in our chairs, and uttered word. He takes a deep breath, exhales slowly, and after a moment of deliberation, continues:

> Look, these Bob Geldof and Live Aid, and all of these concerts have their incredible intent of what they wanted to do. I just, however, think that here is where the fine line comes on accepting those kinds of events, the efficacy of them, how effective they are. Do they make any difference? I say yes and no. Artists, for example, are often paid huge sums to come to these events, and help spread the message, they may expect a three-bedroom suite at a hotel, they

> may drink a lot, and possibly other things to make themselves feel relaxed, that sort of thing. So, for me, those events, what they were trying to affect, I don't think they reached the optimum of what they could have done. I don't discount, however, the intent. For instance, I don't think at in the first Mandela concert [46664] there was very much literature passed out, I don't know how available condoms were. We all saw on television the performances, and I personally, but again here is where anyone's interpretation of a song will be diverse as ever, I hardly thought any of the songs had any relation to a person changing their behavior. For me, that was a huge PR exercise for many different things, but as I said, I appreciated the intent.

He furrows his brow for a moment in contemplation before his expression settles into one of sincerity and earnestness. Readjusting his position in his seat and leaning forward to place his hands together on the desk, he goes on.

> What we do is different, we try to inspire you to do something, or even just to go back to your community and knock on that HIV-infected person's door next door and say "hi, how are you doing? Here's a bowl of soup", as opposed to ignoring them. One doesn't have to do what we are doing to make a difference; it could be the smallest gesture. The bigger campaigns at least managed to get people talking about AIDS. It's still a major problem in many rural areas for people to talk about HIV and AIDS; they can't get it off their lips. Actually, forget rural areas, when my brother died, my mother had for years told everyone he died of cancer. She couldn't say he died of AIDS-related complications. Anything on that scale that gets more people to put the letter and words on their lips in order to get a conversation started was invaluable at the time.

* * *

South Africa is a country in which singing is intimately intertwined with history, culture, and identity. As a consequence, an implicit challenge emerges when writing a book with the title *Songs of the South African AIDS Crisis*. What applications of song are to be discussed in these pages? While this has been a question that has guided much of the writing process behind this book, some examples of the application of song and music with the AIDS crisis, such as the 46664 AIDS benefit concerts mentioned above, stand out more distinctly than others. Professor Perry's remarks highlight some of the complexities surrounding applying stadium-sized music performances and celebrity humanitarianism to public health issues with multifaceted and interconnected social, political, and economic determinants, such as AIDS in South Africa. In this chapter, I explore some of those complexities by examining the highly audible involvement of high-profile domestic and international recording artists in music performance-based consciousness-raising efforts, the foundations from which these events drew inspiration, and the broader context of edutainment as an approach to HIV intervention at the height of South Africa's AIDS epidemic.

Edutainment and the Marketing of Health

Edutainment interventions are common approaches to public health awareness across the world. Broadly speaking, these methods present medical and/or social information through entertainment media (Tufte 2008; Singhal and Rogers 2012). Edutainment strategies come in a variety of forms, but two of the most common are the narrative-based approach and the audiovisual messaging approach (Berry 2007; Walker 2022b). The first utilizes the broad appeal of television dramas, weaving its messaging throughout the narratives and dialogues of the program's characters. The program provides a vehicle through which audiences may vicariously experience the health and social issues addressed in the show (Tufte 2005; O'Leary et al. 2007). This approach can also be applied to live or recorded theater productions, such as those discussed later in this book. The second approach capitalizes on the appeal of audiovisual media and live music performances, such as segments of pop music, live concerts, music videos, television and radio adverts, or social media videos, and is largely designed to raise funds and awareness around specific health and/or social issues.

To best understand the use of music and audiovisual media within health and humanitarian campaigning, it is useful to turn first to those who have the most experience in using music to influence behavior. Retail marketing campaigns have been using music to sell products since the earliest days of radio broadcasting (Taylor 2012). Ever since a correlation was made between consumer behavior and profitability, it is within the disciplines of marketing and business that we find a large body of literature on the subject of music and decision-making. The use of music in advertising has been extremely successful; so much so that we barely notice its involvement. However, just as many scholars have warned against treating audiences as passive listeners or viewers (Hall 1980; Askew and Wilks 2002; Cavicchi 2002; Schechner 2004), it is also important to highlight that consumers are also not passive entities that simply absorb messages presented in adverts. People are likely to employ reasoning to determine the credibility of statements made in advertisements, since over periods of time consumers will likely become sensitive to the means by which advertisers assert their influence (Huron 1989). In order to circumnavigate this almost instinctual reaction to new information, marketers must find new ways of overcoming skepticism. Sensorial appeal has proved to be an effective means through which this may be achieved.

Music provides a channel through which to convey messages via affective means and may help to soften verbal cues. As musicologist David Huron highlights, "utterances can sound much less naïve or self-indulgent when couched within a musical phrase rather than simply spoken" (565). Thus, framing messages within music—what he refers to as lyrical language—affords the ideas or proposals held within advertisements a certain resilience to scrutiny or credibility judgments. Indeed, avoiding direct instructions in order to improve their reception is not a particularly new concept. Anthropologist and historian David Kertzer (1988) points to an old Confucian adage, which suggests that rulers should avoid, where possible, giving commands. The reason for this is that direct verbal commands "always bring to the subject's mind the possibility of doing the opposite" (13). While this kind of subconscious suggestion may seem manipulative when presented in such insidious ways in capitalist consumer culture, there are indeed similarities between the use of music in advertising and in health campaigning, at least in terms of the underpinning theories. For example, both forms of campaigning may use music as a way to bring their message to large numbers of people or frame those messages within music to avoid directly telling people what to do. One might easily argue that the entire concept of edutainment is borne out of these same principles.

Research into music and advertising from scholars of ethnomusicology and musicology has sought to analyze the various musical approaches taken by marketers over the years. According to Timothy Taylor's (2012) extensive analysis of the subject, one of the first major forays into musical influence in advertising was in 1962 when Phil Davis, a respected jingle composer, was commissioned to compose a song for Beneficial Finance. Davis explains that

> [t]he lyrics and music of a service commercial, like Beneficial Finance, go beyond the literal. A man may have a pressing financial problem, which may or may not be in the forefront of his consciousness, but from which he basically seeks relief. Literally, this is a serious situation; yet, to write lugubrious lyrics or music would deepen the severity of the pressure. So the musical commercial producer does the inverse. He composes happy lyrics and music that suggests to the listener a possible happy solution to the problem. (Davis, cited in Taylor 2012, 108)

What is interesting to note about this extract is how similar this conception is to the models applied in modern health campaigns, including some of the most famous examples of pop music humanitarianism from the 1980s that will be discussed later in this chapter. Despite dealing with issues of poverty, hunger, or disease, campaign messages are often hopeful and typically set to music that reflects this in order to create some kind of positive energy or effervescence. As a result of its mass appeal and seeming ability to transcend region, class, language, and other boundaries, NBC Executive Frank A. Arnold noted in the early 1970s that music was the great common denominator in media broadcasting (Taylor 2012). This would appear to be one of the pivotal aspects of music in all forms of campaigning—its mass appeal and some potential explanations for this have already been outlined in Chapter 3.

An early study on music and behavior in advertising entitled "The Effects of Music in Advertising on Choice Behaviour: A Classical Conditioning Approach" (Gorn 1982), is considered to be one of the first studies in the field. It found that products and brand messaging would be viewed more favorably if associated with some object or thing that is met with a positive response (Johnson and Wagner 2011). Concordantly, the participants' intent to buy increased while listening to music that they enjoyed, while the opposite effect was observed while listening to music that they did not enjoy. A third dimension is added when dealing with edutainment or other health initiatives insofar as they must not only strike a balance between standing out and appealing, but must do so while not overshadowing the medical information or messages within the music.

It is clear that music has the potential to offer certain influential components to marketing campaigns including entertainment and memorability, as has been the case since its use in early radio. But in the decades since, music has taken on a more sophisticated set of roles in advertising. It grants marketers access to a wider range of emotional appeal through sensory stimulation. Appealing to the senses can give brands and products more aesthetic and emotional value (Hultén, Broweus, and van Dijk 2009). The more an idea or object can be associated with sensory input, such as certain sights, sounds, or smells, the easier it is to create personal and emotional connections to it. Since we are often not overtly aware of these marketing techniques, these values may seem true, innate, and appealing. Dubbed cultural synesthesia, this phenomenon describes associations that are made between objects and values and are strengthened through a combination of multiple sensorial cues (Howes and Classen 2014). A useful example of this can be found in the sensorial association of burning incense with Buddhist or Christian prayer as an olfactory sensory trigger for the spiritual or the divine.

These associations can become powerful triggers in creating mass indices around a brand or product. Such experiences create indexical connections between and among large groups of people and can be highly profitable. Not only are they important for creating a brand, but also in bringing people together around that brand. Though it will be discussed in more detail in the following chapter, it is worth noting a prominent South African example of this here. The contemporary use of songs from the liberation struggle—for whatever purpose—may have the ability to mobilize listeners around sonic memories. These memories of struggle and eventual freedom can be empowering, reminding individuals of prevailing against overwhelming odds. The sonorous oralities tell stories that South Africans can be proud of and help to strengthen the connection between current events with previous resolve and eventual victory (Drewett 2008). Applied to marketing, those sounds help to create a community around a particular product, campaign, or idea through common association. Many of the same techniques used by consumer industries to market their products are applied to the marketing of health and ideas about health.

All of this is to say that the concept of edutainment is built upon principles that have been in use for a long time. And while edutainment as an approach to public health also has a relatively long history—an early example can be found in the influence of the Popeye cartoons on spinach consumption between the 1930s and 1950s—the approaches most readily utilized within the South African AIDS crisis largely developed during the 1990s. It has since become one of the main educational devices used to communicate health information. The goal of such interventions is not simply to raise knowledge and awareness of HIV/AIDS, but to facilitate healthier behaviors through wider social change (Tufte 2008).

Defined by Singhal and Rogers (2004) as "the process of purposely designing and implementing a media message to both entertain and educate, in order to increase audience members' knowledge about an educational issue, create favourable attitudes, shift social norms, and change overt behaviour" (5), edutainment initiatives are not only responsible for the vast majority of South Africa's HIV/AIDS awareness raising but also deal with other pressing social issues such as crime and gender-based violence. The power of edutainment tends to be drawn from its ability to engage with emotional appeals, discuss otherwise taboo topics in public, and role model the kinds of behaviors that lead to improved health outcomes (Cousins 2009).

Health communication scholar Thomas Tufte (2005) outlines three major shifts in edutainment development communication discourse since its inception. The first generation are considered the "expert-driven" initiatives, in which social marketing techniques were used to promote a social good. These techniques draw heavily from the approaches to marketing and advertising discussed earlier to "sell" a non-commercial product. The second generation began to pivot toward societal as well as individual change. Rather than focusing specifically on the personal experience of individuals, the inclusion of social structures and collective thought broadened the potential scope and influence of these initiatives and would go on to become an important pillar of edutainment scholarship to come. The move away from the individual toward the social helped to influence the environment in which individual choices are made. By doing so, initiative organizers hoped to create a landscape conducive to behavioral change (Singhal and Rogers 2012). However, the third and current generation of edutainment initiatives attempts to address broader issues, including biases, socioeconomic barriers to the implementation of information, or prejudices. For Tufte (2005), this generation focuses on social critique, challenging inequities, and social change. In the most recent implementation of edutainment, which has remained in a relatively stable incarnation for a number of years, it is understood that a deficit of information is often not at the center of the problem; rather, structural inequalities and deeper societal or community-level problems that hinder meaningful social change must be addressed and resolved.

Similarly, Brazilian educationalist Paulo Freire outlined in an interview what he deemed to be fundamental principles for the development of marginalized communities. He suggested the following: "the need to conquer space, to challenge normative, moral, and social borderlines, and to arrange a critical dialogue on pertinent issues as a pathway towards social change" (cited in Tufte 2005, 167). This approach provides avenues through which questions relating to power, structural inequalities, and human rights can be integrated into edutainment strategies (Tufte 2005).

While much good has come from these initiatives, the methods can still present problems. Perhaps one of the largest disadvantages of edutainment lies in its fundamental link with entertainment itself and by extension the entertainment industry. The reputation of the entertainment industry to promote high-return commercialized material, including popular music, and the idea that entertainment has become the antithesis of learning creates an additional hurdle for edutainment initiatives (Singhal and Rogers 2012). Moreover, edutainment campaigns need to be acutely aware of cultural understandings of play, entertainment, and leisure time. Resistance to messaging can manifest at the reception end as a result of selective exposure, cultural misunderstandings, confusion, and perception (Cousins 2009). This becomes more likely when listeners are identified as passive audiences to media rather than active participants. The connection of edutainment campaigns to questions of power is an important one; it serves as a reminder that fundamental development issues, in this case, HIV/AIDS, should not be treated in a vacuum.

The Legacy of Live Aid in South Africa

Around early November each year in the United Kingdom, when the nights in the northern hemisphere are inching out the evenings little by little every day, the sights and sounds of the local high streets transform. Street lamps and leafless trees are adorned with twinkling lights, novelty snowflakes, and icicles sparkle with reflected iridescence, and the soundscapes of the shopping districts are awash with the unmistakable tones of the enduringly popular Christmas classics. Within this eclectic and disparate repertoire, there has always been one song in particular that stood out to me, even as a child growing up with this annual metamorphosis of public spaces up and down the country. While most of the other songs that make up the annual Christmas collections focus their attention on the holiday or its closely associated meanings of family, Christianity, and the giving or receiving of gifts, Band Aid's "Do They Know It's Christmas?" has deeper layers. With lyrics like "Feed the world, let them know it's Christmas time" and the controversial "but tonight thank God it's them instead of you," the song seems to sit apart from other celebrated Christmas classics. The reason for this is simple: it is not just a Christmas song.

Band Aid was the brainchild of noted humanitarian Bob Geldof. In 1984, the then-lead singer of the Irish punk band the Boomtown Rats, brought together some of the biggest names in the British and Irish musical entertainment industry—including Sting, Bono, Phil Collins, George Michael, and Boy George—to collaborate on a charity single, the funds of which would be used to provide relief from widespread famine in Ethiopia. The result was "Do They Know It's Christmas?" The single was enormously successful, raising over 110 million GBP toward its cause (Kapoor 2013). It went on to become the United Kingdom's top-selling record at the time and is still to this day the second most purchased single in the country's history of record charts, only being outperformed by "Candle in the Wind," Elton John's 1997 tribute to the late Princess Diana.

At the time, *Spin Magazine* noted that "Band Aid's 'Do They Know It's Christmas?' captured the imagination of Britain and America" and characterized it as a "tiny voice raised against an incalculable tragedy" (Guccione Jr. 1986, 6). While a tiny voice is perhaps not the most accurate of descriptions given its success, enduring influence, and sheer weight of star power, it did capture the imagination of millions of listeners. Band Aid's single was one of the first and most financially successful musical collaborations among celebrity recording artists orchestrated to raise global awareness and funds for humanitarian purposes. While a case can be made that George Harrison's "Bangla Desh" (released in 1971) was the first purposefully composed charity single—the proceeds of which were donated to provide relief to the millions of refugees in the newly independent state of Bangladesh (formerly East Pakistan) following the 1971 Liberation War—it was not until the increased globalization and communication technologies of the 1980s that new spaces for celebrity interventions were created (Cooper 2008). It is in this decade that the charity single and benefit concert methods of fundraising for global health and humanitarian causes exploded into the Western consciousness. Some scholars have noted that by the end of the decade, there was scarcely a progressive movement that did not have its own mega-event that drew attention to social or health issues with an intensity that was previously unheard of (Garofalo 2005).

Following the success of Band Aid, Geldoff would invite many of the same artists who participated in the "Do They Know It's Christmas?" single to perform live benefit concerts the following year in 1985, with an even larger collection of superstars, which now involved industry titans such as David Bowie, The Who, The Rolling Stones, Madonna, and Queen. The objective was the same as that of Band Aid: to continue to raise funds and awareness about the ongoing famine. Once again, the concerts proved to be hugely successful, with tickets selling out for the transcontinental concerts at both Wembley Stadium in London and the John F. Kennedy Stadium in Philadelphia.

In addition to sold-out stadiums, the seventeen-hour concerts were broadcast live via satellite to an estimated 1.9 billion television viewers across the world (Baker and Bennett 2022). With the collective star power, support from the entertainment industry, media attention, and tens of thousands of densely packed spectators, the sheer scale of the Live Aid concerts facilitated a significant upswing in charitable donations in the United Kingdom. As sociologist Alison Anderson (1997) highlights, donations to Oxfam more than doubled from 23.9 million GBP to 51 million GBP in the years following the concerts, with the events themselves raising 110 million USD collectively. However, as culturally significant as these events and media were, Band Aid and Live Aid proved to be emotionally powerful yet ultimately transient examples of musically driven humanitarianism. Moreover, the brand became marred in scandal by allegations that an unspecified amount of the proceeds was used to buy weapons for local armed groups, fueling conflict in the region.

Despite their shortcomings, it is difficult to overstate the influence of Band Aid and Live Aid's celebrity-driven mass media approach on celebrity advocacy and philanthropy. The effects were felt almost immediately. Only a matter of months after the release of "Do They Know It's Christmas?," another collaboration of stars, this time gathering in the United States, recorded their own charity single, "We Are the World." This new supergroup included American heavyweights such as Michael Jackson and Lionel Richie, alongside some of the artists who had been involved in Band Aid, and was collectively known as "USA for Africa." With the release of "We Are the World," *Spin Magazine* further noted that "the tiny voice became a booming chorus" (Guccione Jr. 1986, 6), recognizing the influence this new form of celebrity altruism was exerting on popular culture.

The description of the "booming chorus" is fitting in a number of ways. It was of both metaphorical and literal significance. The metaphor of the chorus can allude to the sheer breadth of reach these artists could achieve and the media hype that inevitably surrounded the creation of a temporary supergroup for a one-time charity single. But it is also literal in the sense that each of these supergroups—indeed the phenomenon has become something of a charity single trope—presented themselves singing in unison in a booming choral chorus. Later that same year would see the first foray of international recording artists into HIV/AIDS relief efforts, with Dionne Warwick, Elton John, Gladys Knight, and Stevie Wonder releasing their collaborative cover of "That's What Friends Are For" as a benefit single to raise funds for the American Foundation for AIDS Research. The track hit the number-one spot in the United States and remained there for three weeks.

In his book *Fabricating the Absolute Fake* (2008), media scholar Jaap Kooijman notes that as a teenager at the time, "We Are the World" filled him and his peers with positivity and pleasure, recounting how enthralled he was by the collective star power and altruism of the spectacle. However, he goes on to rebuke the campaign for those very same reasons, arguing that the artists involved in USA for Africa used their status and musical talents to "provide relief with optimism and good cheer" in the face of human suffering (21). While it is true that campaigns like USA for Africa and Band Aid typically provide well-meaning and positive sentiments around situations of global health crises and human suffering, such an analysis is superficial. The point that Kooijman misses is that the feelings he and his peers experienced were very likely intentional, and more importantly, fundamental to the success of the campaign.

Drawing from the experience and expertise of the advertising and marketing industries, such as the strategies applied within the adverts for Beneficial Finance noted earlier in this chapter, the often urgent or dire subject matter of the humanitarian cause is expressed within the charity single in ways that are designed to create a hopeful and uplifting experience. As a child growing up in Scotland, I was exposed to the same optimism and good cheer that Kooijman mentions, as "Do They Know It's Christmas" was played every year during the festive season in shopping malls and other public spaces. Despite the distressing subject matter, the song was not generally associated with human suffering, but with the sentiments of generosity that are so enthusiastically presented around that time of year in the United Kingdom (and indeed the Western world more generally). This is, of course, not to say that my own experience of the song is the only interpretation. Rather, it is to suggest that the often harrowing issues raised through such songs are typically expressed within narratives of positivity.

Kooijman is, however, in good company. Many scholars accuse celebrities of trivializing humanitarian issues and using them as opportunities to improve their own reputations (Kapoor 2013; Nickel 2012; Cooper 2008). While I discuss this particular approach to consciousness-raising in some detail in Chapter 9, for now, it is sufficient to simply acknowledge that the methods used by these campaigns are necessary for the immediate, albeit often fleeting, emotional responses that these supergroups and mega-events pursue. As a result of the successes of these early campaigns, it has become a well-established approach to humanitarian campaigning that seeks to motivate people toward financial donations. And while this success is measured within narrow parameters, the modus operandi for all of the aforementioned campaign events was to raise money, and they did so very effectively.

While international organizations such as the United Nations (UN) and the World Health Organization (WHO) have been implementing strategies to combat disease since the Second World War, and it is also not the first time musicians have involved themselves in philanthropic pursuits, the 1980s supercharged celebrity involvement in global health challenges and paved the way for other initiatives and organizations to incorporate similar methods into their own campaign strategies. This shift was an important one, as it was the first time that ordinary people, who were not normally involved in matters of world health or humanitarianism, were invited to contribute to interventions.

Band Aid and Live Aid marked a turning point in how funds were raised for global humanitarian causes, and some of the world's worst crises were brought directly into people's homes through mass media (Rojek 2012). Band Aid and Live Aid largely became templates for later pop mega-event campaigns that followed. Throughout this book, I use the terms "Band Aid method" and "Live Aid method" to refer to the use of celebrity musician interventions in both pre-recorded and live venue settings, respectively. The financial success of these supergroups has resulted in a wealth of similar concerts and music video humanitarian campaigns over the past thirty years, including several reincarnations of the original 1984 single.[1] In South Africa, this came in the form of the 46664 AIDS benefit concerts.

The 46664 Concerts and Breaking the Silence

A somewhat frail-looking and elderly man makes his way slowly to a podium at the center of the stage. His entrance is met with rapturous applause, and his likeness, emblazoned across the vast canvases that stretch across one side of the stage, casts a characteristically warm smile across the entire crowd. Nelson Mandela, anti-apartheid struggle hero and first president of the liberated South Africa, begins to deliver his opening message at what will be one of many international Live Aid-inspired music events known as the 46664 concerts. "Let us use the universal language of music to sing out our message around the world." Flanked by an impressive cohort of international superstar musicians, Mandela's words flow through an enormous PA system and reverberate throughout a sea of multiracial faces. The thousands-strong crowd, bathed in a soft orange glow by muted halogen floodlights, responds in an eruption of applause and whistles of approval.

Fear, stigma, and blame cultivated a culture of silence around HIV/AIDS in the early years of the epidemic. The pervasiveness of the silence found it infiltrating the country's social and personal spheres, urban and rural areas, and institutions such as churches and schools (Morrell 2003). This phenomenon, however, was not unique to South Africa, and similar cultural taboos around HIV/AIDS, health, and illness have been noted elsewhere across the African continent and the Western world, most notably the United States (Gamson 1989; McConnell 2020).

This culture of silence is reflected in the experiences of PLHIV across the country, and while it has been discussed earlier in this book, it is worth repeating here to highlight a phrase that is common within the vernacular of AIDS activists: AIDS does not discriminate. During my conversation with TAC activist Fikelephi Dombolo Sithole, who was in her early twenties when she joined the organization in 1999, difficulties in discussing the issue became apparent during a series of events that led to her diagnosis.

> When I was diagnosed with HIV, I was not sick. I was running races with colleagues from work. At that time, I was working at a pharmacy. There was a guy who was selling life insurance policies and things like that. He took me to a private doctor and took my blood to make sure I was healthy. Then he came back to me to tell me that my policy was not approved but there was no reason, he didn't tell me why. When I asked him, he just told me that the policy was denied. Not long after that. I started coughing up blood, so I went for a TB checkup but the checkup came back negative. At that time, there were no counsellors, it was only nurses doing all the work. She asked to draw more blood for more tests but said I'd have to wait for 3 months to get the results. After 3 months, I was really feeling sick. She told me that my result came back as HIV positive and my viral load was 46 million copies, which means that I had full blown AIDS. (Interview with Fikelephi Dombolo Sithole, June 2022)

Fikelephi's experiences not only demonstrate the culture of silence that emerged around the disease but further highlight that these difficulties were experienced throughout a cross-section of South African society. As a virus that is commonly referred to—including in this book—as one that overwhelmingly affects South Africa's poorest communities, Fikelephi's statements act as a reminder that the emerging educated and multiracial middle class of the late 1990s was not immune from the disease or the shroud of silence.

Much of the responsibility for the scale of South Africa's AIDS crisis belongs to the country's early postapartheid government's neoliberal fiscal policies and lack of economic restructuring. However, the ramifications of misinformation and confusion reached beyond the startling AIDS statistics and accelerated social stigma associated with HIV. Since HIV is a serious infectious disease with a high mortality rate if left untreated, fear of infection is an understandable position for those who do not know how to protect themselves, but the fear and silence on the issue had to be overcome for those same reasons. The "break the silence" slogan mentioned earlier in this book is one that seeks to create a climate of acceptance through an audible proclamation of one's status (Morrell 2003). The statement is an act of defiance toward the dominant status quo of silence through highly audible means. Indeed, audibility would become a central theme for AIDS activists in the late 1990s and early 2000s.

One of the most high-profile approaches to breaking the culture of silence came in the form of the 46664 AIDS benefit concerts organized by the Nelson Mandela Foundation. Leaning heavily into the semiotic potential of their association with the former president and liberation struggle hero (466/64 was Mandela's prison number while incarcerated on Robben Island) as well as the international influence of celebrity musicians and performing artists, the concerts were primarily concerned with combating silence by making as much noise about AIDS as possible. The first concert was held on November 19, 2003, in Cape Town's Green Point Stadium. One of the main slogans used by the 46664 campaign was "awareness and education through entertainment," making explicit their goals of raising awareness and their specific approach to the crisis.

Drawing inspiration from the celebrity-driven mega-events of the 1980s, the concerts attracted some of the biggest international and African singers and musicians. Indeed, it is clear upon a cursory glance that these concerts were very similar to Live Aid in particular, given that the lineup for the first 46664 concert bore striking similarities. Many of the musicians who had been involved in Live Aid had also provided their services to the 46664 concert. In fact, some medical ethnomusicologists have noted that the two campaigns "presented an almost unsettlingly similar approach" (Barz and Cohen 2011, 12). In short, the 46664 concerts became South Africa's humanitarian mega-events.

The 46664 concerts were planned for several months prior to the performances, unlike the famously rushed organizing of the Live Aid performances—in which Geldof would announce bands before they had confirmed their attendance. The funding was sourced from media companies and major corporate donors including Coca-Cola, MTV, and Warner Records (Barz and Cohen 2008). The first 46664 concert was able to present a cross-cultural performance composed of African and Western popular musicians including Bono and the Edge from U2, Brian May and Roger Taylor from Queen, Eurythmics, Beyoncé, Youssou N'Dour, Yvonne Chaka Chaka, Ladysmith Black Mambazo, and the Soweto Gospel Choir, to name only a few. These performances were staggered so that there was a largely even spread of African and Western performances throughout the concert.

Thematically, the concert adopted the approach of the shout, as noted earlier. The concept of making as much thematically interconnected noise on the subject of AIDS in South Africa was threaded throughout the performances. Refrains of rhythmic chanting to the slogan 46664 were frequently encouraged to bind the audience together in a sonic and synchronized display of solidarity against the scourge of AIDS but also to reinforce the associations between Nelson Mandela's unrivaled moral authority and the need to raise one's voice and break the silence of AIDS. This was an important step, given that the risks of speaking openly about HIV had led to the brutal murder of AIDS activists, as noted in Chapter 1. Despite his age and ailing health, Mandela appeared in person at many of the 46664 performances. By juxtaposing the metaphors of war, struggle, and triumph, the former ANC leader strengthened the connections between the struggle for liberation and the struggle against AIDS, even going as far as to suggest that while he had spent twenty-seven years in jail, those who were suffering from AIDS in silence were figuratively in jail themselves. The concerts, he indicated, were their chance to be freed.[2]

Allusions to HIV were developed throughout the event. The participation of Brian May and Roger Taylor without Queen frontman Freddie Mercury—who had died of AIDS-related complications in 1991—presented a powerful visual representation of loss. Anastasia, whose vocals were filling in for the absent Mercury, capitalized on this thematic framing with the rhetorical apostrophe "you are the champions" during one of the band's most famous tracks, "We Are the Champions." Further, specially composed songs for the event included "The Call," written by May. This song both challenges all of the men in the audience to "be a man," implicitly referencing the rhetoric of AIDS activists that real men talk about AIDS while simultaneously alluding to the telephone campaign in which members of the public could dial the number 46664 and donate to the Foundation. Finally, the timing of the first event, which was held a matter of days before World AIDS Day, clearly represented the agenda of the concert.

Many of the organizers and performers within the 46664 concerts had not only been a part of the flurry of celebrity concerts and charity singles of the 1980s but had also actively been involved in the international movement that utilized their music and celebrity status to vocalize opposition to the apartheid regime in South Africa. One of the most high-profile expressions of musical opposition to the regime—notwithstanding Paul Simon's controversial *Graceland* collaborations—came in the form of the supergroup Artists United Against Apartheid. Organized by Steven Van Zandt, the group included industry stars such as Bob Dylan, Run–DMC, Peter Gabriel, Bono, and Bob Geldof, among others.

The artists involved in the track also pledged not to perform at the Sun City resort, which, due to dubious claims to be part of the so-called independent Bantustan of Bophuthatswana, was not subject to the UN-imposed cultural boycott of South Africa. Their single, "Sun City," while not as commercially successful as "Do They Know it's Christmas?" or "We Are the World," still grew popular enough to join the ranks of popular anti-apartheid protest songs such as Stevie Wonder's "It's Wrong" (1985), Eddy Grant's "Gimme Hope Jo'Anna" (1988), Peter Gabriel's "Biko" (1980), and Labi Siffre's "(Something Inside) So Strong" (1987).

Later, in 1988, the Nelson Mandela 70th Birthday Tribute Concert was held in London's Wembley Stadium—in the same venue as Live Aid three years later—and was subsequently characterized as a more political version of the era-defining mega-event, but with the goal of raising awareness of the subjugation of Black South Africans under the apartheid system rather than raising money for alleviating hunger in Ethiopia (Denselow 1989). Many of the aforementioned protest songs appeared in the setlist for the concert, but the powerful symbolism of the show lay in the nonattendance of the man for whom the celebration was ostensibly held. Mandela, still imprisoned after being transferred from Robben Island to Pollsmoor maximum security prison, was a conspicuous absence.[3] The process of raising awareness was highly successful, with many outside of South Africa becoming aware of Nelson Mandela and the struggle for liberation (Evans 2014).

The 46664 concerts drew inspiration from the mega-events and supergroups of the 1980s, in part due to the overlapping narratives and connections between the AIDS crisis, the anti-apartheid movement, and the explosion of celebrity advocacy during that decade. It has been claimed that over a billion people viewed the opening concert in Cape Town and raised millions of dollars for the cause of HIV/AIDS prevention and awareness (Barz and Cohen 2011). In light of this, 46664 is widely regarded as a success, but as was the case for the other mega-events, this success is measured through the narrow lens of views and funds.

Proponents of the concerts argue that their enormous scale and the international reach of the artists provided the kind of exposure to a public health crisis that it otherwise would not have had. As such, they served as an important milestone in addressing the silence that had emerged around the subject of AIDS. In terms of raising awareness of the issues, it is difficult to argue with this sentiment. The Live Aid method has proved itself time and again to be effective at getting people's attention. There are few better examples of a space that one might expect to elicit musical effervescence than a mega-concert of this scale. From the booming sound systems that amplify rhythm and pulse, soaring vocal lines from charismatic superstars, to messaging that exudes an ecstatic altruism, the 46664 concerts had the full weight of the music industry and corporate sponsorship at its disposal to create a celebrity-driven musical spectacle not seen since the 1980s.

Critics of the concerts, however, have argued that though many allusions to HIV/AIDS were made, there was little meaningful engagement with PLHIV or information regarding prevention from high-risk behaviors, as "actual discussion of AIDS were generally limited to spoken interludes during the concert" (Barz and Cohen 2011, 12). Given that South African national HIV/AIDS prevalence in 2012 had risen to 12.2 percent of the population from 10.6 percent in 2008 (the year of the final 46664 concert)—a real-world increase of 5.2 million new infections (Shisana et al. 2014, xxiv)—it is reasonable to suggest that success, defined only in terms of funds raised, may not translate into successful prevention.[4]

Given the limited time within the concerts dedicated to discussing HIV, it is not difficult to determine that the 46664 concerts fell into one of the more striking pitfalls of this kind of celebrity engagement, that is, oversimplification. For the most part, celebrity advocates, though informed of their charity's goals, are not trained experts in their chosen field of philanthropy. This lack of professional knowledge has led some scholars to argue that the oversimplification of complex issues into slogans or sound bites only serves to present a false simplicity of reality.

> The "analysis" rests in the language of rock songs, Hollywood, and Ronald Reagan. The world is painted in black and white and good is pitted against evil. Nuance is inevitably lost. Historic experience is disregarded. Celebrities provide their followers with easily understood, morally couched messages, but the process of development is much more complex. (Dieter and Kumar 2008, 260–1)

Moreover, one of the most significant deficiencies of the 46664 concerts was their reliance upon an approach that was popularized in the 1980s, what Tufte (2005) referred to as the second generation of edutainment intervention strategies. This approach focused on presenting the problem to communities in the belief that raising awareness alone would be sufficient to resolve it. But as I have already noted earlier in this chapter, at the time of the first concerts in 2003, edutainment initiatives had already developed more nuanced understandings relating to the influence of structural inequities, socioeconomic critique, and social change on health and humanitarian issues.

Fundamentally speaking, a deficit of information was not at the core of the AIDS crisis, and an argument can be made that the audiences were not active participants in the edutainment intervention, a critical methodological misstep. In short, the 46664 concerts applied a model from a different era to a public health crisis with deep and complex historical, social, political, and economic determinants. Raising awareness and funds with a mega-concert did not address—or indeed try to raise awareness of—the fundamental issues of structural violence, inequality, gender-based violence, postapartheid macroeconomic policy, or lack of economic restructuring that are significant factors in HIV infection risk. If they had, then perhaps there would be more cause to consider their implementation of the Live Aid method in keeping with more contemporary edutainment approaches as outlined above.

Moreover, while the concerts appear to have had all the necessary components to facilitate musical effervescence as outlined in Chapter 3, the kind of manic creativity that is the hallmark of musical effervescence failed to materialize. As noted by Barz and Cohen (2011), the purpose—a core property of this phenomenon—was poorly integrated into the event, resulting in associated states of synchronicity and an affectively charged musicking environment that served little function outside of its entertainment value for the participants and boosting the humanitarian credentials of the performers. Furthermore, the superficially participatory elements of the event provided few opportunities for organic connections to be made between those involved in the event.

Very few of the songs were related to HIV/AIDS, and no instructive literature or condoms were distributed. Notwithstanding the remaining members of Queen, few international performing artists who participated in these concerts had previous experience in HIV/AIDS awareness and prevention or any meaningful connection to the cause. As a result, the purpose associated with each artist's decision to perform at the concerts is difficult to determine. There is also much skepticism in the literature on celebrity advocacy surrounding the motivations for superstars to become involved in such highly publicized humanitarianism, a sentiment shared by Professor Perry in the opening of this chapter. Indeed, there is no data that examines the reasons behind the participation of the audience, rendering any claims about their purpose for attending speculative at best. Moreover, given the largely presentational nature of the live performances, with celebrities far removed from the audiences and shielded by security, opportunities for creating important connections with the audiences that underpin the music, synchronicity, and embodiment were of limited scope and thus resulted not in musical effervescence but rather the animated responses of music in the moment.

This is, however, not to say that the 46664 concerts provided no benefit to the struggle against AIDS in South Africa. Just as Live Aid was able to fleetingly harness the affective qualities of music to motivate individuals enough to donate money to a cause, so too did the AIDS benefit concerts draw from those same principles to promote the importance of talking about the health crisis. To repeat a quote that opened this chapter from the late Jimmie Earl Perry, "anything on that scale that gets more people to put the letter and words on their lips in order to get a conversation started was invaluable at the time."

Despite their flaws, Band Aid and Live Aid indisputably started something of a revolution in humanitarianism, providing a mold for future mass media, fundraising, and musical intervention to galvanize support for a cause. They set a precedent for a now familiar campaign model of music videos and live concerts that forms the contextual backdrop for understanding the many audiovisual health campaigns that followed, some of which are discussed in this book. The 1980s was the beginning of a new age of global campaigning, one in which social issues, popular music, and celebrity endorsement became inseparable. But while these methods deployed in the health crisis through the 46664 AIDS benefit concerts did have their role in breaking the silence around the epidemic, they did not actualize the potential of musical effervescence to facilitate new conceptions of social relations and realities. As a result, important critiques have highlighted the limitations of such approaches. To find examples of where this phenomenon did emerge, we can turn to groups of individuals for whom purpose and participation manifest more readily. Some of the most powerful examples of musical effervescence come from within the activism of the Treatment Action Campaign (TAC) that are analyzed in the following two chapters.

Notes

1 In South Africa, the anti-crime campaign "Shout," along with a collection of local artists, has released two music videos: one original song of the same name in 2012, as well as an earlier cover of John Farnham's "You're the Voice" in 2010. In 2014, Bob Geldof created "Band Aid 30" which released a cover of "Do They Know It's Christmas?" to raise money to fight the Ebola outbreak in West Africa, and more recently, African artists from across the continent have come together to create a music video for the "No Xenophobia" campaign in response to the 2015 violence against foreign nationals in South Africa called "No More."

2 It would seem that the juxtaposition of associations was successful, given that Professor Jimmie Earl Perry referred to the events and the "Mandela concerts" during our interview quoted at the opening of this chapter.

3 Although he would be transferred again later that year to Victor Verster prison near the Cape Winelands town of Paarl, where he would stay until his release in 1990.

4 This potential rift between monetary success and awareness of a specific issue can be further exemplified by Band Aid 30, Geldof's latest incarnation of the Band Aid franchise, to raise funds to combat the 2014 Ebola outbreak in West Africa. The venture raised over one million GBP in the first few minutes of its release (Jeffreys and Allatson 2015). However, some expressed discontent with how the song represented Africa and questioned the need for another Band Aid. Indeed, West African artists formed their own supergroup, Africa Stop Ebola, to tackle the outbreak. While Band Aid's main focus was to raise funds, Africa Stop Ebola sought to both reduce the spread of the virus as well as prevent further outbreaks by circulating health information on Ebola transmission. Each campaign contributed to the Ebola prevention cause, the fight against Ebola prior to Band Aid 30 was shamefully underfunded, but it is clear that the two initiatives have very different approaches and respective goals. For Wildenthal (2013), effective humanitarians not only "forge powerful yet evanescent bonds with their donor publics through the media" as celebrities often do but also "carry out actions requiring great personal bravery and endurance; and they rely on cooperation from local people at the sites of the humanitarian crisis" (105). Africa Stop Ebola was the result of artists reaching out to people within their own region and actively engaging with West Africans in their own languages as part of a locally based initiative, though it is important to note that there is little data on the efficacy of the Africa Stop Ebola campaign.

6

"Wake Up! Demand It! Sing!"

Song and Struggle in the Treatment Action Campaign

Chanting. Dancing. Whistling. The sound of jubilant ululation rings out over call-and-response cries of HEALTH OVER PROFITS! Standing together outside an imposing building, the low mid-winter sun forms a looming shadow over the small crowd. T-shirts emblazoned with the slogan HIV POSITIVE adorn almost every individual as the scene pans its way across the collection of activists. Through the clapping and shouting, a melody begins to emerge, growing in volume as more people join the familiar tune. The small group of women who had started singing together are now accompanied by dozens more, filling out the choral harmonies of the well-known anti-apartheid struggle song, "Thula Sizwe." Marching together in front of the US embassy in Cape Town, the energy of the song washes over the crowd as they move in step to the implied meter of the music. The smiles and songs belie the gravity of the situation faced by the individuals in the video, but such is the nature of South African struggle songs. In times of greatest hardship, they have provided pillars of hope and community support.

I rub my eyes and check my watch. It is after midnight and I am sitting at my office desk, still staring at my computer screen at a historical snapshot of Cape Town, South Africa, in 1999. I am able to do this as a result of the thorough digitizing and curating of thousands of hours of audiovisual material made available by the Community Media Trust (CMT) and the University of Cape Town in the form of the CMT AIDS Archive (nd). The material meticulously documents the TAC's journey from a small collection of committed and desperate protesters to a national powerhouse of political activism. After many hours spent combing through the videos of the archive, I became aware of parts of my body moving to the rhythm and pulse of the songs and chants, sympathetically mirroring—albeit to a much smaller degree—the movements of those figures on the screen. My body was drawn, partially, briefly, and anachronistically, into the lived experience of that moment in history. Such are the occupational vulnerabilities of working with the creative outputs of passionate and determined people motivated by purpose, urgency, and illness.

It took a great deal of time to settle on the title of this book. The broad range of topics covered in these pages made pinning down something concise and relevant, yet meaningful and eye-catching, quite the challenge. The title *Songs of the South African AIDS Crisis* primarily attempts to capture the essence of the many manifestations of music within the country's ongoing battle with HIV. But no title can perfectly express everything that an author hopes to say. Indeed, a title may index some aspects of a narrative more readily than others. I believe that the title of this book and the topics discussed over the next two chapters are perhaps the most strongly connected. For those of us who have engaged with the history of South Africa's struggle against HIV, some of the most influential and impactful songs of the South African AIDS crisis are those that have been, and continue to be, sung by the TAC.

Much has been written about the TAC, given its highly influential role in the battle against AIDS in South Africa. Scholars from across the world have provided biographical representations of the group (Geffen 2010), explored its influence on global health politics (Mbali 2013), examined the relationships between the organization's methods and the previous struggle against apartheid (Robins 2008), and provided a contemporary examination of the group more than twenty years after its founding (Powers 2020). But within this wealth of description and analysis, there is one glaring omission. Throughout this vast literature, there is almost no substantial discussion relating to one of the most powerful tools for motivation and mobilization deployed by the TAC, their use of culturally resonant and emotionally charged songs.

As Geffen—one of the few to even give a cursory nod toward the subject—writes *in Debunking Delusions*, when TAC members come together "you can bet that songs will be composed with tunes borrowed from the struggle against apartheid" (2010, 190). This tangential and offhand remark from Geffen is indicative of the degree to which the literature has ignored the TAC's use of songs as vehicles to meet its goals. However, it simultaneously highlights something of crucial importance to understanding the TAC, its processes, and methods. Geffen, a former TAC member from early in the organization's history, notes that every single time members are together, they sing. Indeed, not just randomly chosen songs or popular tracks, but new songs with tunes from the old struggle repertoire, creating connections between the TAC and the struggle for freedom that helped propel the organization to its current position as South Africa's most influential AIDS advocacy group.

Through discussions with former TAC members and months spent digging into the archive, a different version of the well-documented story of the TAC began to emerge, one in which songs play a central role. In this chapter, I discuss the goals of the organization and the methods that were applied in order to meet those goals. I explore the previously ignored, yet liberal use of songs in their struggle for access to AIDS medication. In doing so, I highlight the crucial role played by musical effervescence, through the use of culturally resonant songs, in the effective mobilization of communities and individuals across previously entrenched racial, class, and ethnic divides that contributed considerably to the TAC's success.

Government Responses and AIDS Denialism

Founded in 1998 by former anti-apartheid activist Zackie Achmat and close friends, the TAC's modus operandi in the early days was to draw attention to the health crisis that was silently ravaging the country. The primary motivation for their activism was the lack of public access to highly active antiretroviral therapy (HAART)[1] that could turn HIV from a death sentence into a chronic, yet manageable condition. While I have already briefly noted the vast literature on the topic of the TAC, and it is certainly not my intention to reinvent the wheel on this matter, it is important to ensure that the discussions related to their use of songs are presented within the appropriate historical framework. Any discussion of the TAC must be situated not only within the endemic structural violence outlined in Chapter 2 but also in the context of the early governmental responses to the emerging crisis. As such, a little more history is in order.

The South African AIDS epidemic began to become visible in the ailing years of the apartheid regime in the late 1980s. This was a time of social and political instability and intensified state-sponsored political violence against the movement for liberation (Powers 2020). The emergence of the epidemic at this pivotal moment in South African history would have two interrelated effects. The first effect was that the ailing apartheid government and its democratic successor would both underestimate or otherwise ignore the growing health crisis. The second was that the campaign for treatment access, spearheaded by the TAC, would emerge from a deeply entrenched and very recent culture of struggle against injustice and human-rights-based activism.

In the early days of the TAC, there was a prevailing consensus among its members that the nascent government of the new South Africa was supportive of their work and that the responsibility for making HAART available in South Africa lay with the multinational pharmaceutical companies and their willingness to either reduce the prices of their patented products or to allow licenses for the manufacture of low-cost generic versions. This belief can be observed in the protest outside the American embassy in Cape Town described earlier, as well as previous interactions with government officials, such as Achmat's meeting with Dr. Nkosazana Dlamini-Zuma, the then Minister of Health. The minister responded positively to an invitation—likely made with some degree of jest—to lead a TAC march to demand price reductions from drug companies.

This consensus can also be identified within the thematic material presented through the various songs that accompanied the TAC marches during this time. In the opening vignette to this chapter, the TAC activists sing a reimagined version of the anti-apartheid struggle song "Thula Sizwe," translated from isiZulu to mean "Consoling the Nation." The message of the song is addressed to a grieving nation, but with lyrics such as "Thula sizwe, ungabokhala" (Be still, country, do not cry), it implores listeners not to mourn for fallen comrades who have been brutalized or killed by the apartheid security forces. It then preaches that God is helping Black South Africans to fight for their freedom, "UJehova wakho uzokunqobela" (Jehovah will conquer for you). The main lyrical themes of the song are support and encouragement at the loss of life and personal freedoms (Kritzinger 2013; Walker 2021a).

With such strong parallels to the experiences of PLHIV, the song was easily molded to present the TAC's message. However, the TAC activists do not sing about uJehova fighting for them; instead, they sing "Thabo Mbeki wakho uzokunqobela." The inclusion of the then newly elected president of South Africa, Thabo Mbeki, as someone who will fight for the rights of South Africans, is a clear indication of the TAC's early faith in the government to support their cause. Mbeki would continue to feature in the activists' songs, but the nature of his inclusion would shift significantly as the AIDS crisis unfolded throughout his presidency.

While South Africa's state-sponsored AIDS denial would peak under the leadership of the country's second democratically elected president in the early 2000s, the national government's mismanagement of the impending AIDS crisis began almost immediately following liberation, during the Mandela administration. While other African governments began to address the emerging sub-Saharan African HIV/AIDS crisis as early as 1986 (Senegal) and 1990 (Uganda), the South African government's response was not only delayed but blighted with controversy. Between 1995 and 1997, South Africa's first postapartheid administration suffered a series of staggering embarrassments early on in the narrative of HIV/AIDS in the country. The most notable were the overpriced theater flop that was *Sarafina II* (McNeill 2011) and the so-called miracle cure Virodene, which under scientific scrutiny turned out to be nothing more than a chemical solvent. Both of these debacles contributed to growing discontent among advocacy groups regarding the government's handling of the epidemic.

In 1995, the Department of Health commissioned a theater production with the goal of raising national awareness of HIV/AIDS. Internationally recognized playwright Mbongeni Ngema was consulted on the subject of penning a sequel to the immensely popular anti-apartheid musical *Sarafina*. Ngema was awarded a 14.27 million ZAR tender to implement the production (Fourie and Meyer 2010). Despite the enormous cost of the proposed production, the project was approved by the Minister of Health. The inflated price raised questions about the legitimacy of governmental oversight. Indeed, it later became apparent that the Department of Health had sent notice of tender to only a handful of theater companies, some of which were given little time to respond (Lindfors 2021). The department received only two proposals: one from Opera Africa, estimating a total cost of 600,000 ZAR, and Ngema's 14.27 million ZAR proposal. Despite mounting concern from the ANC's political opposition and the national media, the government remained defiant in its support of the project. Following accusations of mismanagement, the relationship between the government and South African civil society, particularly AIDS activists and organizations, began to deteriorate (Fourie and Meyer 2010). This was one of the first signals of a developing AIDS orthodoxy within the government, and the National Department of Health in particular, with anything outside of that orthodoxy slandered as "counter-transformationalist, disloyal, or even racist" (Fourie and Meyer 2010 94). A consequence of this kind of rhetoric was that it positioned AIDS advocacy groups as enemies of the government, rather than legitimate critics.

The audibility of the accusations of corruption regarding the cost, tender, and lack of oversight of *Sarafina II*, coupled with its designation as an unauthorized expenditure after investigation by the public protector, and subsequent shelving under the Mbeki administration, marked what critics would come to describe as a governmental position of corrupt and reactionary AIDS anti-intellectualism or anti-science (Geffen 2010; Mbali 2013). Unfortunately, the *Sarafina II* fiasco would only serve as an indication of what was to come in the following years, as the division between consecutive governments and AIDS activists continued to grow. In her discussion of AIDS and politics in South Africa at the time, Schneider (1998) explains that the immediate effect of conflating political allegiance and public health was to undermine and damage the non-discriminatory aspects of the national AIDS response. *Sarafina II* illustrated that the government understood that edutainment (in this case musical theater) was emerging at the forefront of HIV/AIDS education in South Africa, while simultaneously sidestepping accountability relating to the poor implementation of HIV/AIDS awareness and prevention programs.

By 1997, the country was grappling with its next AIDS scandal. Virodene was an ineffective AIDS medication developed by H. F. Verwoerd Hospital technician Olga Visser and her husband Jacques Siegfried "Zigi" Visser. The developers were awarded a 3.7 million ZAR research grant for their work despite little evidence to suggest that Virodene could in any way combat AIDS (Fourie and Meyer 2010). The mishandling of government funds, however, would be the least alarming revelation during the Virodene scandal. A report from the University of Pretoria and the Gauteng Health Department would later show that the main compound within Virodene was actually the industrial solvent Dimethylformamide (DMF) and proved beyond reasonable doubt that the so-called cure was harmful to humans. DMF is a chemical solvent used in the production of, among other things, plastics, pesticides, and adhesives, which the European Union Dangerous Substances Directive classifies as toxic.

To make matters worse, it soon became very clear that the researchers had deviated radically from standard protocol and ethical norms for conducting human trials. Not only had they misinterpreted the so-called anti-viral properties of the chemical but also moved to human clinical trials without ethical clearance or any prior experience in toxicology (Mybrugh 2009). As was the case with *Sarafina II*, Minister of Health Nkosazana Dlamini-Zuma defended both the actions of the Virodene developers and her department. For much of the South African media at the time, in supporting researchers who announced results without peer review and who conducted unauthorized and unethical human trials on the seriously ill, the minister's continued support was tantamount to announcing that mitigating the AIDS crisis was less of a concern than party loyalty and pride (*Mail and Guardian* 1998).

While these scandals set the tone for the state's responses to AIDS, their place in the history of the HIV epidemic is often overshadowed by the events that followed. Perhaps the most instrumental figure within this contentious period was deputy president (1994–9) Thabo Mbeki, who later took over office from Nelson Mandela to become South Africa's second postliberation president (1999–2008). As communication and media scholars Fourie and Meyer (2010) note "Thabo Mbeki's controversial views on AIDS and his two governments' objections to, and foot dragging on, treatment rollout have rendered him infamous amongst the local and global AIDS community, scientists and most of South African civil society" (1). If anything, with an estimated 330,000 preventable deaths attributed to policies of denial in Mbeki's government between 2000 and 2005 (Chigwedere et al. 2008), Fourie and Meyer's comments are quite understated. The controversial views include opinions on the links between HIV and AIDS that are exemplified in a speech given at the 13th International AIDS Conference held in Durban. He stated

> extreme poverty is the world's biggest killer and the greatest cause of ill health and suffering across the globe. [. . .] As I listened and heard the whole story told about our own country, it seemed to me that we could not blame everything on a single virus. (Mbeki in Decoteau 2013, 80)

While Mbeki's identification of poverty as a core issue driving the AIDS crisis was accurate, his denialist rhetoric on the causal link between HIV and AIDS was reactionary and dangerous (Fourie and Meyer 2010). Moreover, the new administration came with a new Minister of Health, Dr. Manto Tshabalala-Msimang, who would claim her own place in infamy among South Africa's AIDS activists. Echoing Mbeki's skepticism of the scientific consensus on the link between HIV and AIDS, she criticized the use of ARV therapies, suggesting that their toxicity may be more harmful to patients than AIDS itself (Nattrass 2012).

The enduring slogan "break the silence of HIV/AIDS" noted in Chapter 5 was unveiled during the same 13th International AIDS Conference and continued to be a hallmark of AIDS activists throughout the crisis. But despite AIDS messaging dominating South Africa's public health discourses and mass media, and due in no small part to the manner in which the subject was dealt with by the Mbeki government, reluctance to openly discuss AIDS would continue to manifest itself in homes, classrooms, and places of work for many years to follow (Morrell 2003; Visser and Sipsma 2013).

There are a number of possible reasons why the epidemic was overlooked in the early years of the new South Africa. The nature of the virus, as a slow-acting attack on the body's immune system over a number of years, may have misled many into believing the problem was not an urgent one. To be sure, after only a brief period of majority rule, the prospect of facing a national health crisis that disproportionately affects Black South Africans would have been difficult to accept. The Mbeki administration maintained that a government-funded HIV/AIDS treatment program would be too costly and ineffective, despite evidence to the contrary illustrated some years earlier in the form of Brazil's public sector ART rollout initiative. As Brazilian anthropologist Joao Biehl (2004) has noted, Brazil proved that AIDS medication could not reasonably be withheld from citizens of the developing world.

Given his relative muteness on the subject since leaving office, it is difficult to know Mbeki's true motivations behind his vehement denial of HIV/AIDS. This, of course, is not helped by his fervent rejection of his government's AIDS dissidence while in office and avoidance of directly stating his position on the matter. Nathan Geffen aptly refers to Mbeki's tendency to sidestep such issues as "obfuscatory waffle" (2010, 48). We can, however, glean some understanding from what he did say while in office. For Mbeki, the AIDS epidemic seemed to be connected strongly to "dark continent" discourses and prejudicial views of "African sexuality" (Arnfred 2004). In 2001, Mbeki opened the World Conference Against Racism with some remarks that helped to illustrate his position. He blamed racist views of Black people as carriers of disease.

> Thus it comes about that some who call themselves our leaders . . . take to the streets carrying their placards, to demand that because we are germ carriers, and human beings of a lower order that cannot subject its passions to reasons [. . .] Convinced that we are but natural born, promiscuous carriers of germs, unique in the world, they proclaim our continent is doomed to an inevitable mortal end because of our unconquerable devotion to sin and lust. (Mbeki in Arnfred 2004, 10)

At face value, Mbeki's claims seemed to hold at least some credibility; after all, apartheid had dehumanized and economically exploited Black South Africans to a staggering degree. After hundreds of years of brutal repression, the ANC still certainly held the moral high ground. Mbeki argued that the Western scientific consensus of the causal relationship between HIV and AIDS, and particularly its categorization as a sexually transmitted infection, was rooted in "deeply entrenched white racial stereotypes of black Africans" (Mybrugh 2009, 2).

These views were likely significantly influenced by the timing of the epidemic: the moment of rebirth for the South African nation (Posel 2008). Mbeki held that in order to overcome the problems left by colonialism, African solutions had to be found for Africa's problems (McNeill 2011). Once again, at face value, were it not for the terrible cost in human life that resulted from it, he could be forgiven for seeking locally sourced solutions. However, his deeply held convictions concerning race, colonialism, and liberation led to extreme short-sightedness in the face of a growing health crisis. By focusing so resolutely on what became known as Mbeki's African renaissance, the highest office in the land became blind to an overwhelming scientific consensus around the cause and effects of HIV.

Moreover, this approach ushered in a revival of traditional African practices that, in some cases, were openly at variance with international medical conventions and indeed the ANC's own proclamation to uphold equal rights for all (Arnfred 2004). One example of this was his endorsement of female virginity testing as HIV prevention, a practice that was not only medically dubious but also reinforced existing gender inequalities. Scholars have noted the significant burden of responsibility implicitly placed upon young women by virginity testing to control the spread of the virus, while remaining silent on the responsibilities of men (Arnfred 2004). For McNeill (2011) this "was an attempt at the decolonisation of consciousness; an endeavour to foreground African-initiated science and question convention" (118). Steps such as this not only encouraged harmful practices but compounded into a climate of confusion around HIV/AIDS transmission and prevention. Mbeki and his government's refusal to commit to comprehensive ART rollout was the result of what has been noted as his inability to "dissolve," rather than merely expose, racial dichotomies (Arnfred 2004, 8).

It is likely that the scale of South Africa's AIDS crisis could have been mitigated if governmental responses had followed scientific consensus. The signification of the epidemic (Treichler 1987; Sontag 2013) pushed policy toward disastrous results. The government's actions and attitudes toward the grim realization of South Africa's HIV/AIDS problem ranged from the underestimated and miscalculated to the criminally mismanaged. For Visser and Sipsma (2013), as a result of the racist politics of South Africa's recent past, the Mbeki administration in particular underestimated the scale of the crisis and prioritized economic and political issues over and above the growing epidemic. The confusion wrought by institutionalized denial of an increasing global, regional, and national problem led not only to the delayed availability of treatment options but also engendered doubt in the minds of a dying population. Despite the failings of the Mbeki administration, however, it would be wrong—as many scholars have done—to lay all responsibility at the feet of Mbeki and Tshabalala-Msimang.[2] Cracks in the government's response to the AIDS crisis, as I have noted previously, began to emerge very early on in the new democracy's history.

A Luta Continua (The Struggle Continues)

The confusion wrought by the missteps of two consecutive administrations saw a growing population of increasingly ill individuals with no access to ARV medication and without clear guidance on the most effective approaches to maintain their health. Into the vacuum of leadership on the subject of AIDS stepped a series of civil society organizations. While the TAC would rise to distinction, the organization was not the first AIDS advocacy group to operate in the new South Africa. Organizations such as the National Coalition for Gay and Lesbian Equality (NCGLE), founded by Achmat and Simon Nkoli, the National Association of People with AIDS (NAPWA), and the AIDS Law Project (ALP), all of which Achmat was involved with to some degree, had all been operating to promote LGBT and PWA rights prior to the founding of the TAC.

The TAC's approach drew from well-established marketing methods—such as those outlined in Chapter 5—and coupled them with the energy of public demonstrations. They built their brand by drawing the attention of the media through various publicity-grabbing ventures such as overtly and unashamedly illegally importing affordable generic versions of medications to reduce opportunistic infections brought about by AIDS (Mbali 2013) and Achmat's high-profile refusal to take ARV medication unless it was available to all. This was the catalyst that prompted former president Nelson Mandela to visit Achmat. During one of these meetings, Mandela wore a TAC HIV POSITIVE t-shirt and further highlighted the international recognition that the TAC was beginning to build when he noted that "people far beyond our borders are aware of the principled stand that he [Achmat] has taken" (Mandela cited in Lewis and Blankenberg 2011).

What set the TAC apart from other activist organizations of the time was the speed at which the group created a national social movement. This can largely be attributed to the methods the TAC deployed to present their message. As Robins (2008) describes it, the TAC "deployed global discourses of science, medicine, liberal rights and social justice together with grassroots mobilisation" (101). The result was a potent mix of rights-based rhetoric, biomedical knowledge, community mobilization, and moral imperative. As it became clear that the Mbeki government was not going to support a national HIV/AIDS prevention and treatment plan, the TAC took to the streets to start bringing this issue to the attention of the general public in the manner in which the original small group of members—many of whom were political activists during apartheid—were most familiar with, through the kinds of rights-based activism rooted in the struggle for liberation.

The TAC's reliance on the anti-apartheid lexicon was—and continues to be—rooted in strong community-like ties, trust, and powerfully symbolic gestures. By aligning itself with such powerful cultural and political symbols, the TAC was able to achieve two important outcomes. The first was to avoid being labeled as a conservative White social movement by its detractors (Robins 2004). The second was to utilize rhetoric reminiscent of past injustices to mobilize large numbers of South Africans across racial, ethnic, and class divides through marches, public demonstrations, and civil disobedience campaigns (Robins 2008).

The organization had all the necessary components for cultivating musical effervescence at their disposal. The group's purpose was strongly associated not just with human rights (which would have been a powerful impetus by itself) but with life and death, creating a palpable urgency among members of the TAC who were infected or affected by HIV. Song and singing, as hallmarks of liberation culture, presented ample opportunities for collective musicking while immersed in the symbols rich in political meaning cultivated over years of opposition to South Africa's minority rule, including, but not limited to, the right fist held high *Amandla!* salute, struggle songs and dance, and referring to one another as "comrades" (Grebe 2011). This multi-sensorial actualization of previously applied iconography could revitalize powerful affective associations with struggle and triumph, while collective musicking provided the foundation for participation, synchronicity, and social intimacy. Given the success of the liberation struggle in the form of recently acquired political freedoms, the knowledge that these methods previously bore fruit nourishes forms of manic creativity that envision social realities in which PLHIV are free from the threat of violence and ARV medication is available to everyone in South Africa.

Singing Can Say Things Better

While their approach to achieving their goal of a national AIDS treatment program was multifaceted and encompassed a range of activities, one particular element was consistent throughout every aspect of their activism: singing. During a discussion with Nkhensani Mavasa, a former TAC activist, she noted the importance of songs within the TAC's movement.

> Singing is very important starting from the beginning of the protest, in the middle and also in the end, right the way through. Singing says a lot in TAC, hence even the songs that we sing, we're not just singing the songs just for the sake of, it's a message that we are conveying. Even if maybe it's a meeting among ourselves, we sing those songs that will encourage some people. That will be, even bringing education to other people. Because even in our treatment workshops or our council meetings or branch meetings, we sing those songs, other people, they're not going to understand what you're saying or hear you by just sitting them down and talking to them, but singing, conveying the message, they can easily understand what you're teaching them or what you're saying to them. (Interview with Nkhensani Mavasa, August 2022)

The TAC utilized the didactic properties of musicking within South African cultures to create avenues through which health information could be sensitively yet effectively introduced to local communities. These didactic qualities draw from the connective and affective properties of songs described in Chapter 3, altering spaces and relationships in order to facilitate a culturally appropriate exchange of knowledge. Participants in the TAC's community health programs bring with them their own, often long-standing perceptions and significations of health and illness. By tapping into culturally resonant methods of engagement, the activists largely mitigate the negative associations of Western biomedicine with colonial exploitation and global north-south hegemony.

Similar experiences of singing within the TAC's meetings and discussions occupied a central place in many of the conversations that I had with another former activist, Fikelephi Dombolo Sithole. She recounted how singing together helped those who were more reserved or inhibited to become involved through songs.

> There are some people, they don't prefer you to talk too much. They prefer to just sit there, but by singing you can convey a message without saying a word to that person and singing can say things better, more than the way you can try to explain to a person. You find that if you're trying to explain to a person can turn to you confusing that person, but by just singing, the person can relate and interpret and you know, say a lot of things from that one song. So, singing has been a culture of TAC in protest, in a meeting, in conferences. (Interview with Fikelephi Dombolo Sithole, June 2022)

Nkhensani and Fikelephi's words bear striking similarity with those shared by Sifisi Ntuli, a former anti-apartheid activist. In the documentary film *Amandla! A Revolution in Four-Part Harmony*, he notes the power of songs to communicate meaning from person to person.

> A song is something that we communicate to those people who otherwise would not understand where we are coming from. You could give them a long political speech—they would still not understand. But I tell you: when you finish that song, people will be like "Damn, I know where you niggas are coming from. Death unto Apartheid!" (cited in Hirsch 2002)

These shared sentiments expressed by the activists in different but related contexts speak to the powerful emotive and communicative effects that music has been observed to have. The application of singing to convey meanings is indicative of a shared understanding among the participants who utilize such songs that they can transcend ordinary linguistic limitations and instead function in the emotive and affective realms of communication. As I have already noted in Chapter 3, if speech or rhetoric were able to effectively communicate every aspect of our humanity, then by virtue of its lack of utility to our survival, it is unlikely that we would ever have developed our capacity for creating music, and even less likely for it to have endured to become an integral component of every culture across the world. The use of songs in the context of communication among the TAC members is a powerful real-world example of this. It is also worth noting that many of the songs that comprise South Africa's immense repertoire of liberation songs are designed to communicate on this affective plane, whether through lamentation, solidarity, or motivation. This is perhaps one of the reasons why they have endured long after their ultimate goal of national liberation from White minority rule was achieved.

This property of collective singing was highlighted again later in my interview with Nkhensani. Speaking of the practical applications of song within the TAC, she noted how singing together as one facilitated conflict resolution within meetings.

> So singing has been a cool thing within TAC, not just out on the marches. If we were in a meeting and there were a lot of disagreements with no way forward, you find that just pausing and having a song, that can refresh people's minds, that can even assist in making people come back to focus, then the discussion can start moving in the right direction. (Interview with Nkhensani Mavasa, August 2022)

During the TAC meetings, singing together helped to overcome differences of perspective or opinion. The deadlock of debate was refreshed through song and social intimacy. Her words express how songs can cut through the messiness of superficial disagreement to reveal commonalities and redirect the energy of the collective toward a shared purpose, goal, or belief—a fundamental component of musical effervescence. Communal music-making—and the effervescence that may follow (particularly during TAC meetings, which were often characterized by their effervescent atmospheres)—connects individuals together, coupling them through musicking the way Huygens' pendulums were coupled together. And like Huygens' pendulums, the group will sympathetically synchronize, sharing not only space and time, rhythm and pulse but also mood and perspective. The call-and-response patterns of South Africa's struggle songs encourage participation as the sonorous harmonies so characteristic of the repertoire engender social harmony within and among the TAC activists. As such, the emergence of musical effervescence within the TAC meetings provided the opportunity for social and cognitive recalibration within the groups.

She continued to express the vast applications of singing within the organization, indicating that songs were composed to express the ambitions of what the members hoped to achieve or to promote individuals to higher positions within the group.

> Songs will prepare the mood, prepare the minds of people, making people to be in the focus of everything that is happening, lots of people will come with their song and will sing their song and the song will send a message about our struggle and what is it that we want to achieve in that congress or that march or that meeting. And sometimes you can even lobby for the kind of leadership you want. Create a song because you can sing and mention the name of the person that you're going with without getting bogged down in argument about why

> they want this person to be in this position. You kind of lobby, try to engage with other people through songs. (Interview with Nkhensani Mavasa, August 2022)

The communicative properties of song not only helped to present new ideas, but as Nkhensani suggests, the songs would prepare the mood for the coming discussion, paving the way for individuals to receive (and become receptive to) new suggestions and information. Much of this book discusses the processes of musical effervescence within large groups of people, and for good reason. These are the most readily observable forms of musical effervescence. Even within the subject matter of this chapter, the TAC's marches and protests dominate the conversation around the organization's approach and achievements. It would be a mistake, however, to characterize musical effervescence as a phenomenon that manifests exclusively within large gatherings of participants. The sharing of space and time and the associated embodiment of communality can be felt at all levels of musicking when each of the fundamental components is in place (purpose, musicking, synchronicity, heightened affective states, and manic creativity). The TAC's active employment of songs to soothe tensions and create pathways for constructive dialogue highlights the activists' intuitive understanding of these processes.

The Songs Were Their Strength

It may have become clear to readers at this point that South Africa's performance-based style of political dissent is one that can be enormously physically taxing. This presented unique challenges for many of the AIDS activists. The sheer physicality of marching, dancing, and singing is strenuous enough for those in good health but poses significant risks for those suffering from AIDS-related complications. In this regard, however, the very acts of physical exertion in communion with others facilitated the resolve to continue.

During my conversation with Fikelephi, she touched upon the strength that communal singing can provide.

> Emotions were high because most people were dying of opportunistic infections that occurred during that time when ARVs were not yet in place. As much as some of us were not fit to do what everyone was doing at that time, even if you can be at the back of the march, you still want to be there and have your voice heard. Singing those songs together, that was what helped them take then next

> step, and then next one, until the march was over. The songs were their strength at that time. (Interview with Fikelephi Dombolo Sithole, June 2022)

As she notes, many people were dying from opportunistic infections, the manifestations of late-stage HIV infection. At this point, the individual is considered to be suffering from AIDS and is visibly ill. Fatigue and muscle wasting are common symptoms of these latest expressions of the illness. Through shared purpose and the synchronized social intimacy of collective singing, these individuals were provided the energy to temporarily overcome their fatigue and wasted muscles to continue putting one foot in front of the other throughout the marches and protests.

In Durkheim's ([1912] 2008) observations of the indigenous Australian rituals, he noted the propensity for collective effervescence to empower individuals to accomplish forms of action beyond that which could be expected of individuals under regular conditions, noting that within an effervescent assembly "we become susceptible of acts and sentiments of which we were incapable when reduced to our own forces" (209). Despite their physical limitations, members of the TAC who should have been too ill to participate marched and sang with their comrades in visible and audible defiance of both their disease and the indifference of the ANC. Durkheim's description of electricity felt among participants of an effervescent assembly appears to be an accurate description of the energy-boosting properties of the musical effervescence within the TAC marches. In Chapter 3, I noted that this represented a form of human potential energy waiting to be catalyzed into a multitude of as-yet-unrealized forms. This description holds true for many of the TAC activists.

At the heart of such powerful examples, questions arise about how these musical experiences were so transformative for those involved, while other groups who drew from the same repertoire of struggle songs—such as the Venda peer educators noted in Chapter 1—did not cultivate the same kinds of effervescent environments. Important clues can be found in the tactical social marketing approach adopted by the group. The TAC was the first organization to encourage their members to be open and unapologetic about their HIV status. While the principle was clear—nobody should be ashamed to be HIV-positive—the real-world effect of this position was to put themselves considerably more at risk of HIV/AIDS-related stigma and violence. This, coupled with the knowledge that, without access to effective treatment, many of the group members' health would soon begin a decline that would eventually render previously insignificant infections deadly, manifestly increased the urgency of their actions, an urgency that was translated into purpose. While it will be discussed in more detail in the following chapter through the analysis of a more intimate form of communal singing, this urgency—and the fear and anxieties that surrounded it—provided the fuel for a particularly potent form of musically driven effervescence. Indeed, so powerful was this phenomenon that it afforded individuals who should have been too ill to stand, the strength to participate and share their belief that a new social reality of treatment access could be achieved.

Like all feelings and emotions, these flourishes of energy are transient, gradually dissipating with the dispersal of groups, but the optics associated with standing, marching, singing, and dancing in open defiance of both severe illness and a dispassionate government engender powerful forms of political capital that are shared through media and marketing strategies that were designed to capitalize on such symbologies. While singing to share the physical and emotional burdens of AIDS will be discussed in more detail in Chapter 7, it is worth highlighting the decentralizing of suffering that musical effervescence may engender through collective musicking with purpose and the kinds of physical effects that may manifest from manic creativity.

While many of the songs sung at these marches were the same, the ANC and the apartheid administrations were not. Metaphors of battle and fighting replaced literalities. However, while the activists that I spoke to were careful to acknowledge that they did not view the government as the enemy, as was the case in the struggle against apartheid—and this has been illustrated at the beginning of this chapter relating to the early days of the TAC in the late 1990s—some responses of the ANC and apartheid police forces share certain uncomfortable similarities, as highlighted by Nkhensani.

> Some of the tunes were calling for the leadership to say, this is the kind of leadership we want. If you are not that kind of leadership, then get out of our way. So, some of the songs were like, we are ready for the battle, come what may. Even if you claim to hurt us, because sometimes we'd even get arrested or beaten by the police. We'll sing the song and use the tunes that will encourage those who are behind to stay even if we are going to jail. If we are going to be arrested, just do it as in your spirit. Just bear in mind that we are doing this for all of us. Not only for some people, but for all of us. (Interview with Nkhensani Mavasa, August 2022)

The collective singing of struggle songs was used not only to encourage people to remain steadfast in the face of state violence, but also to strengthen emotional and physical resolve to absorb such brutality, if necessary. Affective states of intersubjectivity mitigated the fear of harm to an extent that permitted disobedience. These same principles were applied to even greater threats during the struggle against apartheid, as protesters sang and toyi-toyied in the face of state-sponsored intimidation, violence, and bullets (Michie and Gamede 2013).

During the early years of my research, I traveled to the TAC's regional district headquarters in Khayelitsha. There, I spoke with Mandla Majola, the regional coordinator at the time, who has subsequently gone on to establish the Movement for Change and Social Justice with the University of Cape Town. A lifelong AIDS activist, Majola spoke with passion about the important role that songs have played throughout the TAC's struggle.

> Singing helps us relate, singing tells us to be one, in a song we become one, we connect at an emotional level. When you connect with others like that, you become powerful and with that power you can demand your rights, you can effect change. It doesn't matter what it is, freedom or access to treatment, you use your voice together with others. Wake up! Demand it! Sing! (Interview with Mandla Majola, June 2014)

Manlda's words outline the sense of interconnectedness that manifests through the TAC's communal singing. The power that he spoke of is one that develops through such connectivity. Purpose, focused attention, and bodies entrained through synchronized musicking serve as the connective tissue that bonds the assembly together. I use this metaphor to represent the muscular power of the collective and the importance of musical effervescence and manic creativity to facilitate and direct that power. After all, one cannot apply the strength of the body's musculature without activating its connective tissues (tendons and ligaments).

Interpersonal connections develop rapidly through the process of musical effervescence. Entrained bodies and minds simultaneously invoke the memories and emotions that are bound up within the songs, while newly created meaning emerges to fuel the effervescent assembly. By appropriating the creative outputs of the nation's liberation culture, the involvement of struggle songs and rhetoric creates what Turino (2008) calls mass indices around the TAC's brand through association with sonic memories and emotions held therein. In this sense, the associations of the music are transferred to the new movement, ironically challenging the very same people, the ANC, who were so instrumental in applying those old songs toward overthrowing the previous government.

Nkhensani developed this further during our discussion by drawing connections between the TAC's activism and a particular moment in the struggle against apartheid that inspired a generation of young South Africans to take up arms against the state: the 1976 Soweto uprisings and the now-infamous murder of Hector Pieterson noted in the opening pages of this book.

> So, we would take those older songs because we remember, you can relate our experience to what happened in 1976. Those tunes were very strong in sending the messages. It was telling what people are saying and you would feel that this person is saying something and this person wants to be listened to. There's power in those tunes. They have a message, they are singing that we are not going to give up until we get what we want. (Interview with Nkhensani Mavasa, August 2022)

While the symbolic connections between this moment and the deaths caused by AIDS-related complications have been outlined in Chapter 1, Nkhensani's remarks highlight the sense of connection to the past. More than simply clothing their activism in the ornamentation and rhetoric of the struggle against apartheid, the songs appropriated by the TAC tap into the spirit of defiance and the associated affective resonances that have become fundamentally intertwined with contemporary South African cultural identity. While the lyrics are often altered to sing about the relevant issues, the sonorous aspects remain largely unchanged, resulting in the redeployment of the cultural weaponry that helped to overthrow White minority rule to the new social and political battlegrounds of the AIDS crisis.

An important element of responses to music is how quickly we are able to interpret meaning from them. For psychologist John Sloboda (2010), there is a wealth of evidence that suggests short musical segments, sometimes as short as one second, can elicit both affective (chills, movement, and other pre-cognitive bodily phenomena) and emotional responses. He notes that "such emotions may be 'read off' the musical surface, rather than through deep structural analysis" (503). Thus, even by employing the soundscape of the struggle, the TAC could rely on members of their community to understand the implicit meanings associated with those songs. As Mandla noted during our interview, this provided not only a connection to a wider historical context of the struggle for human rights, but also a sense of motivation and possibility of what could be achieved in their own struggle.

> These songs have a strong connection with the past. We sing the songs of our predecessors and we feel that connection. A connection with the past. Remember

> what was achieved by our elders. Our country has freedom and rights now because of their resolve and sacrifice. Singing those songs connects us to that, spiritually and emotionally. (Interview with Mandla Majola, June 2014)

Mandla's words seem to reference the kind of creativity noted by Durkheim, a creativity through which new conceptions of life may be rendered and revolutions cultivated. By creating connections to the past, the songs act as conduits for this same manic creativity and energy that helped to motivate and mobilize the struggle for liberation. The meanings of the songs emerge from and are bound within their rhythms, harmonies, and melodies, and the new lyrics blend with former associations with contemporary issues to transcend the historical context of their creation. Indeed, the influence of music within many social movements depends less on meanings and associations found within the lyrical content but rather on the relationships created through musicking, including those with the past (Roy 2010).

A powerful example of this was noted during my conversation with Fikelephi. Quite unexpectedly to me, and in mid-sentence, as if it would be more beneficial to show than to tell, a slightly husky, yet beautifully taciturn melody began to flow from her lips. Quietly at first, as if with a sense of subtle self-consciousness one might experience when returning to an unpracticed talent, she began to sing the opening phrases of "Emzabalazweni," meaning "in the struggle."

> Babekuphi lababantu emzabalazweni, emzabalazweni
> Where were these people during the struggle?

(Interview with Fikelephi Dombolo Sithole, June 2022)

Within a few moments, Fikelephi's voice grew louder and her performance more energized. Clapping her hands to her implied beat, she skipped from soprano to alto, call to response, as her voice subtly cracked from time to time through the sheer exertion of attempting to portray all harmonic parts, only to return for a further round of ornate vocality.

> Abahlali babekhona, amahostela ayekhona
> Emzabalazweni, emzabalazweni
>
> Residents were there, there were hostels
> In the struggle, in the struggle

(Interview with Fikelephi Dombolo Sithole, June 2022)

Just as quickly as the rendition had started, Fikelephi's voice falls silent and for a moment she says nothing, her last notes hanging in the air before returning to herself. She explains that the song lyrics reference the 1976 Soweto uprising through the cyclical call-and-response lyrical motif and straightforward questioning: where were you? This song served a dual purpose within the TAC's activism. The first was to remind the ANC government of their role in the struggle against apartheid and the second was to highlight the hypocrisy in their absence from the current struggle for treatment access.

This is an appropriate moment to consider the risks of directing the iconography of the struggle, awash with symbolism of revolution, toward the new administration. Such acts made the organization susceptible to accusations of sedition. After all, these songs and political symbologies were so recently deployed to overthrow a tyrannical government. Indeed, members of the government at the time, most notably ministers of health, accused the TAC of antipathy toward the ANC and seeking power and influence for themselves. However, such attacks had little material impact on public opinion. Since HIV/AIDS overwhelmingly affects those living in impoverished or low-income communities, and given that economic status was still largely divided along racial lines, the TAC was able to challenge accusations that it was anti-Black and simply in opposition to the ANC by motivating members of township communities to march with their cause. Ultimately, the TAC activists unequivocally demonstrated that the performance culture of the liberation struggle could not be controlled exclusively by the ANC by virtue of its claim to be the vanguard of the slow-burning revolution that wiped apartheid into the history books, but rather that it belonged collectively to the people of South Africa.

Throughout many of the interviews that I conducted with current and former members of the TAC, one song in particular was referenced more than any other: "Thina Silwela Amalungelo Wethu." The song speaks of *amalungelo* (rights) and translates to mean "we are fighting for our rights."

> Fikelephi: We used to sing our struggle songs, sizo zabalaza, we were struggling for ARVs but there were many different kinds of songs that we were singing. One we sang a lot was *Amalungelo thina silwela amalungelo wethu*. This song means that we are fighting for our rights because we have a right to access medication, irrespective of what the government is feeling. (Interview with Fikelephi Dombolo Sithole, June 2022)

* * *

> Nkhensani: There was one that was saying [singing] "*amalungelo, thina silwela, amalungelo, amalungelo wethu*," which means we are fighting for our rights. It's not like, for us to have our rights, it not like somebody is like giving us a privilege. I don't know how to put it, but it is our right to get health services. It's our right to be protected, it's our right to have the freedom of speech and all those kinds of things. It was an emotional song. (Interview with Nkhensani Mavasa, August 2022)

* * *

> Mandla: The song "We Are Fighting For Our Rights", you'll hear people singing it at a lot of different protests. It's a song that stakes the claim of why we are here: we are here because we are angry about a particular incident that has taken place in our community, or we are here because we demand justice, we are here to demand our rights. That is an experience felt by us, by our friends, by our comrades, and we feel that support. So, our songs seek to tell our story, to tell people what we are all about. (Interview with Mandla Majola, June 2014)

It is clear from the discussions that the song "Amalungelo" references not only the connections between the TAC and its struggle heritage but also situates the organization's goals within the powerful culture and rhetoric of human rights and social justice. By specifically referencing rights, the use of "Amalungelo" by the TAC activists leaves little room for interpretation regarding their goals. For the TAC, the lack of treatment was interfering with their human rights, the right to life. Not making medicines available was tantamount to killing those who could not afford the high costs of medication and therefore represented a form of tyranny that those who originally sang of *amalungelo* (rights) would not have expected to return to their country so soon after the protracted struggle for liberation. Described as an emotional song by Nkhensani, it was Mandla who elaborated on these emotions, noting the anger and frustrations felt by their perceived lack of justice and indifference from the state.

There is a dignity to "Thina Silwela Amalungelo Wethu." As Majola noted, for the activists, it "stakes a claim to why we are here." But that dignity should not be conflated with morose inaction. As a product of the more militant era of MK and civil disobedience after the Soweto uprising, the expression *thina silwela* (we are fighting), while metaphorical, is representative of the force that was brought to bear upon the government through every available channel, with the powerfully transformative effects of musical effervescence at the core. It is a resounding refusal of circumstance, one that, as noted earlier, could be averted (and eventually was) through appropriate government health policy.

We Filled That Hole with Song

While the concept of community-based therapy will be discussed in detail relating to the TAC choir The Generics in the following chapter, it is worth noting that singing was utilized as a coping mechanism in various contexts and throughout the organization. During a discussion with Fikelephi, she highlighted the importance of songs and singing outside of the previously mentioned highly visible and audible displays of musicking in the marches and protests.

> Songs played a huge part in changing people's lives—not just because it helped us to get what we needed, access to treatment, but because it helped us to feel better at the time. There was a big hole in all of us and we filled that hole with the song. The noise of the gatherings, with the marches, the sit-ins at the department offices, all of it was singing. It brought that hope to people, it was like a light in the dark. I can put it that way. (Interview with Fikelephi Dombolo Sithole, June 2022)

The hole that Fikelephi describes is that of the absence of facilities providing care or support for PLHIV. As she had noted earlier in our conversation, when Fikelephi was diagnosed with HIV, there were few available resources, not just for biomedical treatment but also for counseling services to facilitate her transition into her new reality of a lifelong (and at the time very dangerous) condition. She takes a breath as before, and a lyrical perfect fourth springs to life as the introductory interval of a song dedicated to the TAC.

> uTAC ifikile save our lives, uTAC ifikile save our lives
> Save our lives, save our lives, save our lives
>
> TAC has arrived to save our lives
> Save our lives, save our lives, save our lives

(Interview with Fikelephi Dombolo Sithole, June 2022)

She explains that this song does not simply represent that the TAC facilitated the introduction of life-saving medication but that it provided a holistic approach to the well-being of its members, literally and figuratively saving their lives. The metaphor of filling the empty space within the activists' spirit with the songs and other noises of their activism is emblematic of what many activists experienced as a result of the membership in the TAC. The organization occupied the spaces left by government inaction.

While the sonorous and cultural connections to the struggle against apartheid facilitated motivation and communication, Nkhensani highlighted that these songs provided empathic connections both with those who had come before and those who were in the midst of their present struggle.

> We also relate to 1976 when innocent people were getting killed because of trying to voice out, because of trying to represent other people. They're just assassinating these people. So, you could relate, you know singing those songs makes you relate, you could feel the empathy and the anger and the sorrow and the pain, you know, all those kinds of things. So, some of these songs, when you sing them, you're not going to finish without crying. And some of them, when you sing, you're not going to finish without getting angry. But you try by all means to say, even if you cry, you don't cry in a way that you lose control. (Interview with Nkhensani Mavasa, August 2022)

The deep connections created by singing the songs of the liberation struggle and the expressions of anger, frustration, and grief once again bear a striking similarity to those noted by former MK militants during the liberation struggle. As one former fighter noted in the documentary *Amandla! A Revolution in Four-Part Harmony*:

> Even when we were dying, the feeling was that when people have died, if you mourn them for too long it demoralises your spirit. So as a result, even when we used to go and bury some of our comrades who had been ambushed on the way, we never used to cry, we used to sing. (cited in Hirsch 2002)

The sentiments of needless loss coupled with determination that the loss not be in vain echo throughout the accounts of both the MK and TAC activists, as Nkhensani continues:

> Even then someone is dying, died because they didn't get fluconazole or just the treatment that they were supposed to get for free and then the person ended up dying. I mean, this could have been prevented if we were listened to, if this could have been done. So many people should be still alive today. We are not saying people are not going to die, but not just because people don't have medication. Not because the services are denied, you know? So, every time you sing those songs you have to think of those people who you have seen dying, others are relatives, others are friends. (Interview with Nkhensani Mavasa, August 2022)

Nkhensani's words reflect the new meanings that were being absorbed by the songs as they were sung in this new struggle. While previously they had developed their powerful cultural influence through engagement with the apartheid state authorities, with each unnecessary AIDS-related death, the songs grew more resonant among those who sang them. Their resolve to continue fighting strengthened to ensure the legacy of their fallen comrades. Within these songs can be found a history of collective action, struggle, dignity, perseverance, and bittersweet victory. Perhaps Nkhensani summarized the influence of songs within the TAC best toward the end of our discussion with the following thoughts: "The songs, the singing, it's been a part of TAC always. In my world, in the world of TAC, and to all of us. I hope it stays like that because it means a lot and it says a lot."

The TAC did not redeploy the songs of the liberation struggle simply due to the convenience of proximity. The communicative, motivational, and therapeutic aspects of singing together provided an effective tool that, coupled with the prominent position of songs across South Africa's cultures, the recent memory of state tyranny, and the resolve to overcome it, ensured that the nascent AIDS advocacy group would have an extensive and powerful range of tools at their disposal.

While the wounds of South Africa's recent past remained open and in a climate of mistrust, stigma, confusion, fear, and blame, the TAC was able to harness the affective, connective, and emotive properties of the country's songs and wider cultural expressions to bring people together across racial, ethnic, and class boundaries to fight for PLHIV. Musical effervescence was employed at all levels throughout the organization and facilitated mobilization, communication, and community-based therapy. The sonorous and melodious battle cries of liberation vibrated through the demonstrations, Durkheim's electricity creating palpable connections between individuals. In such situations of heightened affective states of synchronicity, musical effervescence binds collectives together, or as Mandla put it earlier in this chapter, "in a song, we become one."

Struggle songs, when used by the TAC in the context of HIV/AIDS awareness, treatment, and prevention, take on what communication scholar Mark Mattern (1998) would describe as a pragmatic role. He describes the pragmatic form as occurring when "members of one or more communities use music to promote awareness of shared interests and to organize collaborative efforts to address them" (29). While Mattern's theory of pragmatic musicking is conceptualized in terms of political awareness, the term is applicable still to the social struggle of HIV/AIDS awareness, not least due to the political history of South Africa's struggle songs and the high-profile legal battles between the TAC and the South

African government. Fundamental to the pragmatic use of arts in action is the coming together of people, whether communities, subcultures, and so on, in some level of shared commonality to address issues broader than those of the individual. Within the TAC's various applications of song throughout its organization and activities, musical effervescence provides a framework for engendering the transformation of individuals into a cohesive and collective force of pragmatic musicking.

As I worked my way through the events documented within the CMT archive and related materials, I found myself observing the first Stand Up For Our Lives rally outside the national parliament buildings in Cape Town. On that bright Valentine's Day—February 14, 2003—the TAC leaders spoke passionately about the new civil disobedience campaign that was being implemented to compel the government to engage meaningfully with the group. But one speaker stood out from the rest. In a striking and deeply saddening moment of contrast within the archival footage, an energetic young man addresses the crowd of TAC activists and supporters through a microphone. His speech crackling with distortion from the audio equipment, the passion in his voice is palpable.

> How can I sing a love song, when my sweetheart is dying!? How can I sing a love song, when my brother is dying!? How can I sing a love song, when my mother is dying!? South Africa, now is the time to stand up for your rights! Treatment plan now! (Cited in Lewis and Blankenberg 2011)

Darting from one side of the stage to the other with animated and exaggerated movements, Edward Mabunda's words and energy stir the crowd, who respond with whistles and yells of approval.

> We're continuing! We're going forward! We're together! We're going to beat it! We're the victors! We're going to run like lunatics! We're going to kick like horses! We're together, we're going to beat it! We're going to beat it together! (Cited in Lewis and Blankenberg 2011)

The scene fades and is followed by the same man speaking to the camera from a hospital ward in Johannesburg, but he is almost unrecognizable. His energy has disappeared and he is visibly ill. The striking contrast between the energetic young man passionately engaging a crowd of hundreds of activists and the weak, pale, and emaciated individual struggling to speak presents a distressing and personal image of the suffering and loss wrought by AIDS in South Africa. In April of that same year, Edward Mabunda died from AIDS-related complications.

Mabunda's passionate address to the crowd at that march offers a powerful representation of the TAC's struggle for HAART at a time when HIV infection was tantamount to a gradual death sentence. "How can I sing a love song?" symbolizes this pain. It is unfathomable to sing of love at a time of such needless loss and tragedy. Instead, the TAC sang of hope, action, determination, unity, human rights, and justice.

Notes

1 HAART refers to an early form of ARV medication that was available in many developed economies when the TAC was formed. Despite its name, HAART is less effective than current ARV medications, and the term has largely been supplanted by TAC activists in favor of ARV or ART.

2 For a list of scholarship that has pointed the proverbial finger squarely at the Mbeki administration, see Nicoli Nattrass' *The AIDS Conspiracy: Science Fights Back* (2012), Nathan Geffen's *Debunking Delusions* (2010), Fourie and Meyer's *The Politics of AIDS Denialism: South Africa's Failure to Respond* (2010), and Mandisa Mbali's *South African AIDS Activism and Global Health Politics* (2013).

7

"Songs That Speak to the Shock of the Loss"

The Generics HIV-Positive Choir and Psychosocial Healing

One of the primary purposes of this book is to highlight the numerous ways in which songs and singing have been applied to the South African AIDS crisis. Throughout these pages, I document a variety of approaches, but perhaps some of the most widely recognizable come in the form of choral singing. There have been a number of high-profile AIDS choirs that materialized during the height of the epidemic. One of the most widely recognized is the Siphithemba group. Emerging from an HIV/AIDS support group at the former McCord Mission Hospital in KwaZulu-Natal, this choir has toured across the world and has been the subject of extensive anthropological and ethnomusicological study—much of it conducted by Austin C. Okigbo of the University of Colorado (Okigbo 2011, 2014, 2016; Okigbo and Ezumah 2017). Other high-profile choirs include the Thembeka Choir, a group that emerged from HIV-positive patients and staff of Durban Hospital (Black 2019). However, one choir that has garnered little attention, despite their significant influence on the direction of the AIDS crisis and their collaborations with international recording artists, is the TAC's very own HIV-positive choir, The Generics.

The TAC's high profile within the narrative of the epidemic has, in my opinion, inadvertently led to a situation in which many scholars unintentionally overlook The Generics as merely an extension of the TAC's wider activism. And while it may be true, to a certain extent, that the choir's activities constituted one aspect of the TAC's public engagement strategy, the lack of scholarly attention paid to this group of passionate and determined individuals sits discordantly with the significant role they have played in achieving the wider goals of the organization.

The TAC is well-known for its use of songs within its marches, sit-ins, and civil disobedience campaigns. Many of the members already had significant experience singing together with others in church choirs, youth groups, or at ceremonial social gatherings known as *imigidi*, but it was not until 2001 that the first official choir, The Generics, was formed. The name was chosen to draw attention to the group's commitment to lobbying the South African government to make inexpensive generic versions of costly pharmaceutical drugs available to all South Africans through the country's public health system. By 2006, there were many choirs in various provinces across the country, each creating their own songs from the repertoire of the liberation struggle. In this chapter, I focus exclusively on the original group that was formed in 2001.

It is worth noting at the outset of this chapter that collective singing and choir groups have effected social and political change in South Africa since some of the earliest years of European colonization. However, it was not until the codification of racially discriminative conventions into law under apartheid that choirs became increasingly politically active. Indeed, according to Jack Lewis, an activist who was instrumental in both the founding of the TAC and the development of The Generics' studio recordings, the idea of developing an HIV-positive choir was inspired by the political choirs that were active during the apartheid years, such as the Federation of South African Trade Unions (FOSATU) workers' choir, whose members lobbied the political system for improved economic outcomes for Black South Africans.

The songs that are discussed in this chapter can be found as tracks on The Generics' 2001 album *Jikelele: Global Treatment*. The choir's members were individuals infected or affected by HIV/AIDS who devoted their lives to their activism in many forms, including a vast array of creative arts and performances, community engagement, and HIV/AIDS literacy programs. As former member of The Generics, Thembeka Majali, put it:

> Choir members were leaders in their own right. For example, Themba Baleni was the Director of Ikhwezi Youth Drama. His cast, Bulelani Mvotho, Xolani Madesi, Samson Baleni, Zimasa May, Andisiwe whose surname I have forgotten, acted in a number of plays in TAC gatherings. The plays had relevant messages on the prevention of mother-to-child-transmission and they performed other plays about the Treatment Plan. They became members of the choir also using creative arts. Me and Nomfundo Dubula as treatment literacy coordinators gave advice on which songs would be relevant for what event and created the message accordingly. Sindiswa Godwana and Busisiwe Maqungo would advise on what message would be relevant for a certain audience and Nondikho Bango led the

songs and coordinated all the different parts for performance. (Interview with Thembeka Majali, July 2022)

While these songs are immortalized through their digital recordings, it is important to remember that they began, as many of the country's recorded musical activism did during the apartheid era, as local community-level improvisations that settled into recognizable melodies and lyrics in response to various needs or social phenomena. In short, the popular protest music recordings were first sung on the streets (Schumann 2008). The Generics proudly continued this tradition of composition at meetings, marches, and rallies.

Mother-to-Child Transmission Prevention

In the early years of the epidemic, one of the TAC's primary goals was the reduction of child deaths as a result of MTCT of HIV. This occurs when the virus is passed from an HIV-positive mother to her child, usually during pregnancy, labor, or breastfeeding. At the turn of the twenty-first century, a drug known as azidothymidine (AZT) could effectively prevent MTCT; however, due to the political climate of AIDS dissidence outlined in Chapter 6, it was not available in the South African public health system. As a result, the TAC and The Generics prioritized their efforts toward lobbying the South African government to make AZT available in all of the maternity hospitals in the country. This is a theme that is found throughout the choir's repertoire.

The Generics' flagship song of their 2001 album *Jikelele: Global Treatment* shares the same name and makes implicit reference to the availability of AZT in other parts of the world. "Jikelele," originally a well-known Zulu folk song, translates to "around the world" or "globally" in English. The song is originally a Christian prayer to sing the glory of God around the world, with lyrics such as "I love Jesus because he blesses all the people of the world." The choir alter the lyrics to reimagine the song and make it their own.

AZT siyayazi ikhusela abantwana kwiHIV, jikelele
(Jikelele Jikelele Jikelele)

We know AZT prevents babies from getting HIV, all over
(All over, all over, all over)

(The Generics, "Jikelele," *Jikelele: Global Treatment*, 2001)

The choir replaces the references to "Jesus" with "AZT" as the entity that is blessing people all around the world with life, but not in South Africa. As a result, the associated meanings of spirituality, healing, and faith are implied through the music and potentially transferred to the TAC for seeking the life-saving drug for those who need it.

"Jikelele" is a blend of African American gospel and Zulu hymn. It follows a call-and-response pattern throughout, which by its nature can involve large numbers of people in the performance. Within the stylistic inflections that characterize the gospel sound (strong vocal presence, antecedent and consequent structure, lyrics referring to Christianity) can be found numerous themes of faith, and performance elements that can stimulate affective intensities, and engender participation and rhythmic entrainment as outlined in Chapter 3. In his ethnography of African American gospel churches, Hinson (2000) notes the songs of praise sung by churchgoers often evoke intense emotional reactions. The musical events he describes elicit various forms of group participation such as clapping, ecstatic praise, and "calling loud hosannas" (208) among a sea of congregants equally energized by the performance.

During our conversations, Thembeka often recalled the fluctuating emotional environment during the choir's performances, a meeting point of, at times, conflicting affective and emotional states of being.

> We were happy, sad and rejoiced at the same time as we sang what we loved to do. There was an energy, a vibe that we all felt, we were connected to each other and to the people around us. The emotions were so high. People would cry sometimes. Sometimes during the songs, sometimes after we had finished a song. It wasn't always sadness though. It's not easy to explain, but there were these feelings that would appear and fill us with energy. The kind of feeling that makes you want to sing louder and more passionately. Sometimes those feelings made you cry, it made other people cry, because you knew what they were trying to express, but you just sang louder. (Interview with Thembeka Majali, July 2022)

The description provided by Thembeka provides a snapshot of the tempest of emotional energy surrounding The Generics during their rehearsals and performances. With the portrayal of such high-energy interconnectivity with others, the results of which at times led to unrestrained emotional manifestations such as crying and raising one's voice in song, it should become clear that these were transformative experiences for the choir and reminiscent of the kinds of nebulous states of affectively charged euphoria described by Durkheim.

Thembeka's account highlights not only the range of emotional experiences that collective singing facilitated for the choir but also the influence that their music had on those around them. The powerful affective qualities of their performances drew individuals into heightened states of intersubjectivity through which a kind of mutual understanding of their purpose could be not simply vocalized and heard but also felt. As I have mentioned in the previous chapter, the urgency of the TAC's activism provided significant purpose behind each of their activities, generating the kinds of manic creativity associated with musical effervescence. This energy—or vibe, as Thembeka calls it—created a kind of magnetism that drew people toward the performances and galvanized spontaneous support for the group's performances and associated causes.

Similar effects were noted by Themba Baleni during one of our discussions when he articulated the ways in which the choir purposefully drew from evocative local songs—often with semiotic associations with the liberation struggle—to encourage others to join their performances. Through proximity to the messaging, the group could raise awareness for the need for collective action.

> We were popular. People wanted to be around us because we gave the environment a particular vibe, and energy, you know? I think at that time, people, they needed anything that can help them to be fine in their souls because there was a lot of fear of dying and a lot of fear of people losing their lives or families, their kids. We built that connection with other fellows you see. So, we created the songs purposefully as another angle of fighting the epidemic and bringing people together, connecting them as one voice, because the government didn't want to come to the party, they just weren't listening. (Interview with Themba Baleni, June 2022)

In this respect, as in the previous chapter on the TAC, musical effervescence served a communicative role within and beyond the group that transcended conventional linguistic limitations and instead communicated on an affective plane. Throughout my conversations with former members of The Generics, the term "energy" was frequently chosen to describe the perception of an animatedly heightened affective atmosphere. As Themba notes, the choir were able to introduce such energy into spaces in which they performed, not only encouraging others to participate but also maintaining the energetic motivation of the movement and bonding bodies together within it.

The Generics make a few notable alterations to the harmonic properties of the "Jikelele" folk song. The descending call-and-response style is retained but with minor changes to the rhythm of the choir's response. There are alterations in the melodic contour of the main vocal line, in which The Generics' singing largely mirrors the stepwise movement of the original in the opening bar. Rhythmically, however, the two melodies are largely indistinguishable from one another. Furthermore, the two versions of the song are similar in terms of timbre and texture. The main difference between the two versions can be found in the revision of the original lyrics. By retaining the majority of the original song's sonorous qualities, The Generics are able to subconsciously ground their cause within a potent cultural landscape, one which has been deployed in glory to God, in defense of African humanity, and in defiance of White nationalism. This powerful expressive force was then harnessed to propel an appeal to the government to implement a treatment plan and uphold every South African's constitutional right to healthcare and life.

By invoking the name of Jesus, the AIDS activists employ shock tactics in an effort to make their voices more audible and encourage people to listen to their message. Similar efforts are noted among HIV/AIDS peer educators in the old Venda region of South Africa. They elicited mostly shock and outrage from local community members by replacing references to Jesus with condoms in the Lutheran hymn "Jesus Is Number One" (McNeill 2011). The logic is easily followed: Jesus saves, but so do condoms. By likening AZT to Jesus, The Generics are implicitly imbuing AZT with some of the emotions and meanings normally associated with South African spiritual life. These messages of hope and faith are particularly important since, as Okigbo (2011) notes, the HIV/AIDS crisis "created an unprecedented form of depression especially in South Africa's Black community, comparable only to that experienced under apartheid" (295).

The Generics' version of "Jikelele" states its purpose from the beginning, over and above everything else. The track opens with the voice of Thembeka Majali, who states the following:

> This is a call for the national implementation of a mother-to-child transmission prevention program in all the maternity hospitals of South Africa. The song is "iAZT siyayazi Jikelele." (The Generics, "Jikelele," *Jikelele: Global Treatment*, 2001)

The use of such plain and unmediated words makes clear the urgency of the song's message. As Thembeka notes, the movement crossed sociocultural boundaries, resulting in a need to approach the songs using different languages.

> Many of the songs are in isiXhosa, but we wanted to make our audience aware of what the song is about and draw attention. We used English as an international language for that. The arts, songs, poems were used as the art of drawing people's attention because sometimes people express themselves through culture or respond differently when hearing the spoken message. (Interview with Thembeka Majali, July 2022)

The name *Jikelele* is fitting for another reason, as it makes reference not only to the availability of medicines across the world—although not in South Africa—but also to the TAC's and the Generics' international activism. While the act of illegally importing generic versions of the thrush medication fluconazole from Thailand, as noted in the previous chapter, is typically highlighted as one of the more significant forms of transnational activism, The Generics choir also played an important role in garnering international support for their cause. Perhaps the most high-profile example of this can be found a number of years after their recording of the *Jikelele: Global Treatment* album in their collaboration with Annie Lennox's Sing campaign.

The campaign was launched in 2007 by releasing the "Sing" music video and humanitarian anthem, a collaboration between international recording artists (including pop music heavyweights Madonna, Pink, Céline Dion, Gladys Knight, Dido, Anastacia, and others) and The Generics choir. The powerfully emotive imagery and driving rock rhythms sonically merge with The Generics' "Jikelele" recording from their *Global Treatment* album to create a powerful call for international funds to help ease the ongoing crisis (Walker 2022a).

For Themba, Lennox's involvement helped to further international awareness of the epidemic in South Africa to pressure the government into addressing issues of slow ARV medication rollout and access to treatment.

> It was so exciting to work with her as a big artist from overseas. I think she gave that kind of spirit of togetherness of us fighting the pandemic. We were utilizing every tool that we could get to portray to the government that we were really in need. (Interview with Themba Baleni, June 2022)

However, despite the success of the Sing campaign, raising over one million GBP for AIDS advocacy groups in South Africa, the contribution made by The Generics—a fundamental point of contact with South African culture and front-line advocacy in the struggle against the AIDS epidemic—is typically little more than a footnote in the narrative of AIDS activism (see Geffen 2010).

Psychosocial Healing

Themba sighs and pauses for a moment. I have just asked the former activist and member of The Generics to describe the period of struggle for HIV medications at the height of the AIDS crisis.

> Peoples' emotions were all over the place, to be honest. Sometimes people would be laughing and smiling one minute and then crying the next minute. It was a very uncertain time and there was a lot of anxiety. Singing together was one of the ways we used to let some of that emotion out. There was a sense that maybe if these things are too hard to talk about, then we can sing about them instead. Even if you can't find the words, you can pour your pain into the songs and let it go. (Interview with Themba Baleni, June 2022)

Themba's words weighed heavily on his voice as he spoke as if the memories of that era were washing over him once again. They highlight an important quality of song and singing, that of emotional expression and the collectivization of emotional burdens. It can be difficult to articulate severe psychological distress such as that experienced by the AIDS activists during the height of the epidemic. In these moments, The Generics, and indeed the rest of the TAC, stepped outside of spoken language to embrace a more affective form of communication. Such an approach makes sense if, as suggested in Chapter 3, singing emerged from some of our most primal needs to express raw and unbridled emotions. As has been shown in the literature on AIDS in Africa (McNeill 2011), singing provides an alternative avenue through which to express oneself. Themba's account of singing when words fail speaks to the heart of why music can be so profoundly therapeutic: it can be easier to sing what cannot be easily said.

In the repertoire of recordings left by The Generics, there are a handful of songs that particularly encapsulate this phenomenon. One of them is called "Ingaba Senzeni Na."

> Ingaba senzeni na? (Senzeni na?)
> Ingaba senzeni na kuwe Thabo Mbeki? (Thabo Mbeki)
>
> What did we do to you? (What did we do?)
> What did we do to you Thabo Mbeki? (Thabo Mbeki)

(The Generics, "Ingaba Senzeni Na," *Jikelele: Global Treatment*, 2001)

It draws influence from perhaps one of the most well-recognized of South Africa's struggle songs, "Senzeni Na." Sung since the 1950s, it has been compared to the American civil rights song "We Shall Overcome" for its lamenting yet stoic timbre (Michie and Gamede 2013). The single questioning lyrical motif that runs throughout the original "Senzeni Na" is powerful in its simplicity and uncompromising in its tenacity. It simply asks "what have we done?" It questions what Black South Africans ever did to deserve such treatment and dehumanization at the hands of the apartheid state machinery (Lee 2010). The main vocal line laments "what have we done?" before the rhetorical question is repeated twice by the choir's response. The power of this motif is that, despite being phrased as a question, it creates a syllogism that illustrates the absurdity of punishing and brutalizing people based on nothing more than the superficial perceived differences of race (Nkoala 2013). "Senzeni Na" represents a potent example of a non-militant song, both in lyrics and sonorous quality, that still manages to evoke and represent the anger, frustrations, and imperative for change at the moral injustices of apartheid. The track does not openly reference the armed struggle, unlike songs composed from the 1970s and 1980s (when the armed struggle intensified) but became a powerful symbol of resistance nonetheless.

The blurred stylistic boundaries between early struggle songs and church hymns, as outlined in Chapter 4, make it difficult to separate faith and religion from the rhetoric of the liberation struggle. Thus, parallel emotional affordances can be found both in gospel hymns and liberation songs on the one hand, and the revised renditions that are applied to the AIDS crisis on the other. The emotional potency of such songs, coupled with the energy created through group performance, is redistributed into the context of HIV/AIDS advocacy.

Like many songs from the 1950s, "Senzeni Na" "is sad and slow, sung with pathos and humility rather than anger" (Cherry 2015, 228). The vocal performances behind the lyrics of The Generics' "Ingaba Senzeni Na" are expressed in a similar fashion. The woe expressed in "Ingaba Senzeni Na" combines the emotional and cultural resonance provided by the reference to the original struggle song with the grief of the uncertain and harrowing experience of living with HIV in a time when AIDS killed. Themba recalled the burdens felt by each of the members.

> I always remember those days in the choir because, for me, the emotions were there. Because some of the songs were much deeper in terms of trying to put things together for our government to provide ARVs. There were some times whereby the choir would feel much sadder because of the situation of the

> country at that time, because look, there was not that much support for those who were affected by HIV, so there was a lot of worry that people were losing their lives. We had to support each other. The songs, the music itself, drove many people in terms of their sadness and emotions, with being able to face the reality of what was happening in the country, what was happening to their bodies, what was happening to their friends or families. It was tough, it was really tough. Those were heavy burdens, you understand? I think that, without the choir, some people would have been lost, really lost. (Interview with Themba Baleni, June 2022)

For Themba, the choir served as a means through which members could draw from their combined strength as a collective to endure their heavy emotional burdens. The strength that the choir members drew from one another through collective singing was necessary to withstand the emotional toll of being infected and/or affected by HIV without the prospect of treatment. As a collective unit, the choir was able to use those previously overwhelming emotions for more focused purposes. The emotional energies associated with fears and anxieties of what was happening to their bodies (or those of their friends and/or families) were refashioned through collective singing to strengthen their purpose, a key component of musical effervescence. One of the most notable purposes outside of the choir's activism—in which they had to maintain a coherent and sustained approach to their community engagement in the face of state-sponsored misinformation, public attempts to discredit the TAC, and widespread HIV/AIDS-related stigma and discrimination—was to provide support to its members. It provided a collective forum through which to grieve the loss of those who had died before treatment access was achieved. Indeed, as I have noted earlier in Chapter 4, Durkheim ([1912] 2008) notes the similarities of emotional and affective states cultivated during both joyous rituals and collective mourning, observing that both elicit similar intensities of effervescence through different sentiments.

As in "Jikelele," the song opens with a short monologue. In the opening few seconds of the track, the voice of activist Nondikho Bango can be heard saying:

> This one is a special dedication to our president Thabo Mbeki. We are singing this song pledging solidarity with people living with HIV and AIDS, asking government to come up with a treatment plan for people living with HIV and AIDS: "Ingaba Senzeni Na." (The Generics, "Ingaba Senzeni Na," *Jikelele: Global Treatment*, 2001)

By naming Mbeki directly, The Generics employ a method of focusing collective attention—and in this case political pressure—on a single person utilized in much liberation music. Songs such as Vuyisile Mini's "Ndodemnyama" (Watch Out), "Hey Strydom, Wathint'a bafazi, way ithint'imbodoko uzaKufa" (Hey Strydom, now that you have touched the women, you have struck a rock, you have dislodged a boulder, and you will be crushed), and Dorothy Masuka's "uDr. Malan Unomthetho Onzima" (Dr. Malan's government is harsh), have famously been used to openly engage politicians since the early days of apartheid. The Generics were acutely aware of the propensity of songs to both inform and encourage collective action, and the history of this process in action (Anderson 1997; Schumann 2008). Songs would inspire defiance, and the practice of naming politicians and maintaining focused attention on something (or rather someone) tangible would often lead to further civil disobedience and boycotts (Schumann 2008).

Throughout "Ingaba Senzeni Na," there are multiple allusions to "Senzeni Na," as the choir asks "what did we do to you Thabo Mbeki?" addressing the main refrain of the song "what have we done?" directly to the president once again. During our discussions, Thembeka characterized the song as follows:

> It was a message to the country's President Mbeki to talk to pharmaceutical companies such as Pfizer, Glaxo Smith Kline and Bristol-Myers Squibb to reduce the price of expensive HIV/ AIDS medicines and for treatment of opportunistic infections and anti-retroviral provision. (Interview with Thembeka Majali, July 2022)

There is a great deal of irony in The Generics posing this question to Mbeki and his government. The refrain of "Senzeni Na" was originally directed toward the architects and enforcers of apartheid. In this instance, however, the inference is that Mbeki, and by extension the governing party, the ANC, had become the very thing they fought so bitterly to overthrow. This was an intentional move by The Generics. Themba spoke directly to this point during our discussion.

> You know, it's hard to be ignored when there are so many of you and you're all singing those songs that helped to put the government where they are today. That was the first time that had happened, you know, when the people used those songs against the ANC. They were the ones who had helped to create a lot of those songs, or at least make them popular. Just taking that model and turning it around on the government, that was a powerful message back then. We were the first to do that. (Interview with Themba Baleni, June 2022)

The Generics ask "What is our sin? Is it AIDS?" alluding to the lines of "Senzeni Na" that mourn "our sin is that we are Black?."

> Yintoni isono sethu'?
> Yintoni uGawulayo?
>
> What is our sin?
> Is it AIDS?

(The Generics, "Ingaba Senzeni Na," *Jikelele: Global Treatment*, 2001)

But the appropriation of "Senzeni Na" has layers of meaning. The Generics choir is overtly equating their own struggle for life and health with the previous struggle for liberation. In doing so, the group clearly places the Mbeki government squarely in the role of oppressor. Moreover, by calling out Mbeki by name, they are making explicit reference to the president's father, apartheid hero Govan Mbeki, who was often associated with this particular song (Stone 2015). In her doctoral dissertation on South African choral music, Mollie Stone (2015) draws attention to an additional function of naming people directly in song. During her interviews with members of different TAC choirs across the country, a number of her participants speak of the therapeutic qualities of directing anger toward a legitimate source. By referencing his father through "Senzeni Na," the activists reflected the nation's resentments relating to Mbeki's absence during much of the anti-apartheid struggle that manifested into anger at his presiding over an administration of AIDS denial. As a result, activists had no ethical concerns training the cultural weaponry of the liberation directly on him.

"Ingaba Senzeni Na," like many former struggle songs, presents a demand for a fundamental right. In this case, it is the right to healthcare, specifically in the form of the newly developed AIDS treatments that were available in other parts of the world.

> Sifuna AZT (iAZT) Sifuna Biozole (iBiozole)
> Sifuna Nevirapine kuwe Thabo Mbeki (Thabo Mbeki) Yintoni ityala ethu'?
>
> We want AZT (AZT) We want Biozole (Biozole)
> We want Nevirapine from you Thabo Mbeki (Thabo Mbeki) What is our debt?

(The Generics, "Ingaba Senzeni Na," *Jikelele: Global Treatment*, 2001)

Around the halfway point of the song, the volume of the backing vocals drops as the choir softly hums their response melodies while the main vocal line implores the government to talk to the pharmaceutical companies to reduce their prices.

Nceda uthethe no Glaxo
uthethe no BMS athobe amaxabiso

Please speak to Pfizer, speak to Glaxo
Talk to BMS to reduce prices,

(The Generics, "Ingaba Senzeni Na," *Jikelele: Global Treatment*, 2001)

Across the African continent, oral traditions such as poetry and storytelling are often accompanied by humming from the audience members, creating an inclusive performance (Okpewho 1992). Humming during storytelling allows for politically oriented monologues to be spoken over an emotive sonic backdrop (Nkoala 2013) and the same technique is applied by The Generics. The song's dynamics then shift back to the resounding volume of the introduction as the choir challenges for the last time "what have we done to you, Thabo Mbeki?"

Despite their many similarities, however, "Ingaba Senzeni Na" deviates from "Senzeni Na" in a number of ways. The harmonic structure is reimagined from ii-I-V-I into a I-ii-V-I harmonic progression readily found in choral music. The main vocal line, though often imitating the contour of the struggle song, is more embellished and often blends with the choir response in unison or to create harmony. This can be accounted for by two main reasons. The first is due to the use of the isiXhosa language over the original isiZulu, in which the phrase "senzeni na?" becomes "ingaba senzeni na?" with the addition of the extra syllables giving the main melodic line more of a descant rather than antecedent quality.

The second reason is that The Generics borrowed the melodic line from South African icon and singer Brenda Fassie's immensely popular 1997 hit "Memeza," demonstrating the choir's flexibility in drawing from multiple sources of social and cultural resonance. "Memeza" deals with themes of violence and danger, with lyrics such as "Bangitholile abangana xolo bangikhomba ngezibam' nemikhonto," translated to mean "they have attacked us with swords and spears." The track also presents a sense of vulnerability and loss of hope in the chorus with the lyrics "Noma nginga memeza ma Akusizi lutho," meaning "even if I shout, it's no use." As a result, not only is using the melody of "Memeza" practical, insofar as it channels the popularity of the original, but it also synchronizes thematically with the material of "Senzeni Na." Indeed, despite the new melody, the uncompromising lyrical question "what have we done?" coupled with an impassioned and emotive vocal performance from The Generics makes a powerful reference to the struggle song perhaps most recognizable for its lamentation of the suffering wrought by apartheid.

"Ingaba Senzeni Na" is not the only example of a song of healing in the repertoire of The Generics. Another can be found in "Thula Sizwe" (be still nation/consoling the nation). This is a Christian hymn and struggle song that presents an expression of solace while simultaneously articulating themes of battle and conquest. It offers a sense of urgency and militancy that is juxtaposed with themes of consolation and healing in the face of crisis. The Generics' version of "Thula Sizwe" constitutes one of the most overt references to the Christian faith.

With lyrics including "Thula sizwe, ungabokhala, uJehova wakho uzokunqobela," translated to mean "Be still, country, do not cry, Jehovah will conquer for you," the struggle song implores the nation not to grieve for their fallen friends and family by assuring them that a stronger and higher power, in this case, God (*uJehova*), is working toward freedom. Like "Senzeni Na," "Thula Sizwe" is sung with pathos, but within the solemnity is a sense of consolation and resolve. The main lyrical themes of the song are support and encouragement at the loss of personal freedoms (Kritzinger 2013). The Generics' rendition of "Thula Sizwe" is virtually indistinguishable from the original. The only alterations made by The Generics are to the lyrics in which they replace God with the TAC, as well as the inclusion of HIV/AIDS as the scourge to be conquered.

> Thula sizwe, ungabokhala,
> uTAC e wethu uzokunqobela.
>
> Don't cry
> Our TAC is going to conquer for us.
>
> (The Generics, "Thula Sizwe," *Jikelele: Global Treatment*, 2001)

Similarly to "Jikelele," The Generics replace the original reference to God with the TAC. For example, the lyrics "Be still, country, do not cry, Jehovah will conquer for you" became "Be consoled, nation, don't cry, our TAC is going to conquer for us," implying that the TAC is the higher power that will conquer the scourge of AIDS in South Africa. The enemy to be conquered is then made explicit in the following lyrics.

> e HIV/AIDS uTAC wakho uzokunqobela.
> In HIV/AIDS our TAC will conquer for us.
>
> (The Generics, "Thula Sizwe," *Jikelele: Global Treatment*, 2001)

Since the original song was used as encouragement, The Generics' replacement of God with the TAC is not as self-aggrandizing as it may perhaps seem on first impression. The TAC's power comes from its members, those whom it is able to mobilize toward collective action, and thus the reference to TAC is not simply an allusion to the organization, but to the people as a whole who comprise it—it is the people who will overcome. As former TAC activist Nkhensani Mavasa recalls:

> You must remember is that there were a lot of people doing different things in different provinces, each towards the same goals of treatment access and breaking the silence of HIV and AIDS. It's easy to think of TAC as a single organization but it was more than that, there were a lot of moving parts. (Interview with Nkhensani Mavasa, August 2022)

By only altering the lyrics, The Generics are able to make explicit their connection with the struggles of the past. Indeed, during our interview, Themba highlighted the ways in which the sonorous aspects of these songs store affective potential that may be drawn upon for new purposes.

> We were thinking about the songs from the struggle. You must understand, these songs tell a story, there's a narrative deep within them whereby just listening to the music, you know the story that is being told. We wanted to use those narratives for our struggle. Everyone would come out with their ideas as we were singing until we had something that we were all satisfied with. We were creating while we were singing. (Interview with Themba Baleni, June 2022)

While the connections to South Africa's struggle history are discussed in some detail in the previous chapter, it is worth noting here again how the narrative of struggle was woven into the songs developed by The Generics and the TAC more generally. "Thula Sizwe" illustrates the process through which new narratives may be fortified through old stories, as well as the power that can be harnessed from the blurring stylistic boundaries between worship music and struggle songs.

Singing songs from the past can help to reinforce connections between the history of those songs, those who sang them, and the struggles they faced. Thus, songs can be used to share the burden of suffering felt by individuals by placing those worries on the figurative shoulders of the collective. Just as songs such as the solemn "Hamba Kahle Mkhonto" (Go well, Comrade) and the haunting "Senzeni Na" (What have we done?) were often sung at funerals to console those who had lost loved ones and comrades to the armed struggle, those same songs were later used again by everyday South Africans who were once again compelled to fight for their rights. Former TAC Khayelitsha District Organizer Mandla Majola spoke of these historical connections during our interview.

> Many of our songs have an attachment to our past, to the songs that were sung by our elders, our predecessors. That is our homage. What we are experiencing now and what they experienced then, it's the same thing, we were fighting for the right to life. Sometimes we change the songs. We change the words to relate to our present-day struggles. But the people know what that song is, they know the rhythm and the flow, but they change the words. They can tell that this song was a song that has been sung for a long time. (Interview with Mandla Majola, June 2014)

By repurposing struggle songs, the TAC and The Generics could not only sing familiar and comforting melodies and phrases as a collective to soothe the pain brought by the epidemic, the wrath of AIDS, but they could also further tap into the reservoirs of dormant emotional potential contained within them. Viewed through the analytical lens of musical effervescence, the mechanics of the process emerge once again from these encounters. The singers are brought together with a purpose that is related to that of the wider TAC movement but unique, insofar as the choir represents a smaller and more intimate collection of participants. In addition to their activism, the purpose that emerges from their descriptions is to help one another cope with the seemingly insurmountable challenges that surround them through a communal support system. Musicking together with familiar melodies that create connections with past suffering and eventual triumph creates powerful spaces for social intimacy, synchronicity, and resultant heightened affective states. Through this process, powerful negative emotions such as fear, anxiety, and anger may be repurposed into a form of manic creativity that provides a medium through which the singers may conceptualize new social realities in which their struggle, like that of the past, will come to fruition. They may cope with the reality of their current situation through the musical sharing of their burdens and the collectively manifested understanding of a potential social reality in which these burdens will eventually be lifted.

Conclusion

Singing is a fundamentally human action, and, as most anthropologists and music therapists would likely attest, singing through emotional pain is a phenomenon that is about as old as humanity itself.[1] But scholarship is not always necessary to explain what many of us have already experienced, to one degree or another. Songs, at times, can seem like an extension of our emotional presence, to the point that singing or listening to those songs in our hours of deepest emotional burden seems innate, natural, cathartic, and cleansing. During my discussion with Mandla, he highlighted this phenomenon as he touched upon his own perception of the importance of song as a coping mechanism.

> Forget about the struggle, forget about apartheid, forget about AIDS. Just look at Africans. If we have lost someone, one of the ways we deal with the pain, coping with pain, is we sing: songs that speak to the shock of the loss. Song helps us deal with the challenges in front of us, whether it's apartheid, whether it's AIDS, whether it's inequality, the problems in the mines, whether it's unemployment or challenges experienced by young people in schools, one of the ways to deal with these things is by singing. (Interview with Mandla Majola, June 2014)

This discussion of The Generics, and their use of choral singing within the struggle for treatment access, is emblematic of this phenomenon. At a time of fear and anger, the choir redirected their legitimate anxieties surrounding death and personal physical attacks due to HIV/AIDS stigma into a frenetic energy that could be fashioned by group musical activities into a powerful tool for change. The urgency of their situation reinforced the paramount importance of their purposes within a literal life-or-death situation for many of the activists, with little outside support. The participatory nature of the struggle songs in their repertoire facilitated the kinds of affective and emotional experiences and energy outlined by Thembeka and Themba—Durkheim's electricity. The synchronization of bodies and minds could culminate in forms of manic creativity that collectivized grief and suffering, and strengthened resolve to further mobilize for MTCT prevention. During my conversation with Themba, he made explicit this process of turning the burden of HIV infection into a resolve for action.

> People, they had a lot of like mixed feelings sometimes. People were dying, there was so much fear, there was anger and frustration, but at the same time we were like: Okay, we are at least doing something about HIV/AIDS in South Africa. Our voices are being heard by the nation. We need to keep raising our voices. (Interview with Themba Baleni, June 2022)

By appropriating songs from the struggle into a choral choir performance, by its nature an interactive one (Okigbo 2011), The Generics were able to take advantage of the multiple layers of meanings within the songs to not only sing to articulate the TAC's demands within the expressive rhetoric of the liberation struggle, human rights, and divine intervention but also to sing for themselves in the form of collective healing. While it would be easy to focus only on the most public forms of musicking, the experiences of the choir members also reinforce that large gatherings are not a prerequisite for musical effervescence. The detailed descriptions provided by former members are replete with the kinds of intersubjective affective intensities that are the hallmarks of the phenomenon. Moreover, their experiences show that musical effervescence may be felt at varying degrees, depending on the context in which it is cultivated, and highlight that these affective states of manic creativity may be achieved in ways that, though not as immediately observable, remain inwardly powerful. While the public displays of emotionally charged musicking associated with protests that have been discussed in the previous chapter represent some of its most tangible forms, the choir's intimate forms of support and its musical avenues for emotional release and catharsis demonstrate more subtle variations of musical effervescence.

Collective singing and the effervescent qualities of heightened affective states of being provided the framework through which support could be rendered for those who were infected and affected by AIDS by cultivating a musically driven manic creativity through which new social realities could materialize (such as those in which HIV medication is available and stigma against those living with HIV is reduced), and drew global attention to the ongoing crisis through collaboration with international recording artists. While there are, of course, overlaps between the activities and narrative of The Generics and the wider TAC, the choir's story is unique and personal. As Themba previously noted, vocalizing the struggle was instrumental in maintaining the momentum toward the TAC's goals. Large numbers of people could be unified behind the rallying cries or mournful laments of songs that strengthen group identity such as hymns, folk music, or struggle songs (Gray 2004). Moreover, the choir's tacit commitment to redirecting their fears and anxieties as PLHIV toward reaching their purpose afforded their performances a potent manifestation of musical effervescence akin to the urgency associated with the struggle against apartheid.

In many ways, the members of The Generics are part of a lineage of South African singers who have sung out their deepest frustrations and aspirations, not only on the streets in protest but also in solidarity with one another in more intimate settings at a time of social exclusion and ostracization (Kivnick 1990). For the singers of the past, such exclusion was fashioned by the White establishments of the colonial and apartheid states, unable to accept a Black middle class. For The Generics, the stigma of AIDS and the signifiers of bodily pollution conspired to dehumanize them to little more than their illness.

Perhaps one of the most profound moments of my interview with Themba was when he noted the ways in which the connections to the previous struggle strengthened the resolve to continue fighting for their lives and the lives of their comrades. As he put it:

> If we cry, we cry, but we won't stop singing. Our brothers and sisters who fought for our freedom didn't cry, they fought and died, and many mourned the loss, but they kept singing. Those voices never fell silent. Sometimes quiet or sometimes louder, but never silent. (Interview with Themba Baleni, June 2022)

As the TAC's first choir, The Generics sang through their fear, grief, and frustration at a time when AIDS killed in order to effect political change that saw the implementation of a national HIV/AIDS treatment and prevention program. Somewhat ironically for a choir, they are unsung heroes of the TAC's struggle for access to life-saving medication. For their contribution, it is important that they are recognized, and their impact on the country's AIDS crisis is not lost to history.

The TAC provides rich ground for the exploration of the songs of the South African AIDS Crisis and the emergence of musical effervescence, but as I noted in Chapter 1, this book discusses the same phenomenon hiding in plain sight throughout multiple applications of song within the epidemic. The following chapter departs from the discussions of the TAC and moves forward in time to the mid-2000s when Stellenbosch University's ACHAM developed its flagship HIV/AIDS prevention and awareness community outreach program.

Note

1 For a more detailed account of this phenomenon, see Davidson & Garrido's edited collection *Music and Mourning* (2016).

8

Ethnographic Encounters with Musical Effervescence in the *Lucky, the Hero!* Applied Theater Mini-Musical

For eighteen months during the research for this book, I was fortunate enough to be associated with Stellenbosch University's ACHAM as an affiliate scholar. The ACHAM was founded in 2003 on the guiding principle that educational institutions should play important roles in addressing the social problems faced by communities. This philosophy, coupled with research that indicated alarmingly low levels of HIV/AIDS literacy among local farm workers of the Cape Winelands Municipality, led to the development of a dedicated community engagement musical theater program. The goals of these performances were to raise HIV/AIDS awareness, reduce AIDS-related stigma, and encourage knowledge of one's HIV status (Davis 2012). The ACHAM's Educational Theatre Company drew primarily from the influence of songs to achieve their goals. The primary motivation behind this approach came from the involvement of late Broadway musical theater actor and singer Jimmie Earl Perry, who joined the ACHAM as the director of educational theater and creative arts in 2004.

Since their inaugural performances in 2005, the scope of the Educational Theatre Company grew from engaging with local communities in the Cape Winelands to performing across South Africa. From 2013 to 2014, I accompanied the group on a number of performance interventions throughout the Western Cape, Free State, and Mpumalanga provinces. During the time that I was with them, the theater company consisted of six actors—each of whom was trained as an HIV peer educator—an administrator, and a sound technician. Touring with the theater group allowed me to immerse myself in their world, one of purpose, music, humor, and friendship. The focus of my attention was their flagship HIV/AIDS edutainment community outreach program, *Lucky, the Hero!* an hour-long mini-musical theater production directed by Prof. Jimmie (as he was affectionately known).

Lucky, the Hero! was developed as a postgraduate project by now television personality Vicky Davis. Linguistically, the production takes a flexible approach. Originally performed in Afrikaans, due to this being the mother tongue of many Coloured South Africans in the Cape Winelands, performances were also held in English with local vernacular dialogue included in the script in a semi-improvised manner depending on the location of the show. *Lucky, the Hero!* comprises eight scenes that are frequently punctuated by narration and musical interludes. There are three main behavioral outcomes that the show seeks to influence: the reduction of HIV/AIDS-related discrimination, consistent condom use, and HIV status awareness. To help facilitate these goals, the ACHAM draws from its close working relationship with @Heart, a nonprofit HIV testing and counseling service that accompanied the theater group on their interventions to provide on-site rapid HIV testing facilities.

The narrative follows the adventures of a young man called Lucky. Living on the fictional "No Problems" farm—a reference to AIDS denial—he and his best friend Two-Time Tokie have a reputation in the community for having many sexual partners. Upon discovering his HIV-positive status, Lucky experiences discrimination at the hands of his closest friends and is abandoned by a community that is misinformed about how HIV can be transmitted. In response to this, Lucky resolves to educate the people of the farm on HIV/AIDS, safe sex, and acceptance of people living with the virus. Donning a pair of hooded red overalls and dark sunglasses, he sets out to his task under the guise of his newly created alter ego, Captain AIDS-Fighter.

While not participatory theater in the most immersive sense, *Lucky, the Hero!* employs fourth-wall breaks and audience interactions at important thematic and narrative moments. According to Davis (2012), audience participation was incorporated into the script during the development of the show in order to create a sense of intimacy and involvement, as well as to acknowledge the audience's existence and maintain their attention. Notable instances include Two-Time Tokie flirting directly with some of the audience members and in the musical finale, during which the audience is addressed by the entire ensemble cast as being part of the No Problems Farm community.

In this chapter, I outline the methods employed by the Educational Theatre Company that harness musical effervescence to encourage participants to take an HIV test and know their HIV status. Through in-depth ethnographic accounts of *Lucky, the Hero!* performances, I conceptually explore the affective environments cultivated throughout the show that culminate in the grand finale. *Lucky, the Hero!* I argue, presents a powerful example of a process through which musical effervescence may be developed and harnessed into positive health outcomes. While musical segments are threaded throughout the narrative of *Lucky, the Hero!* much of the connections to the main purpose of the performance are cultivated through character development, role modeling, and narrative, and it is the finale in which the significant influence of the song becomes clear. The show ends with a reimagined rendition of Gloria Gaynor's "I Will Survive," a fittingly positive and optimistic send-off and metaphor for surviving through the HIV/AIDS epidemic. By utilizing a multi-modal approach to the intervention, the performance is able to draw from a number of affective and communicative approaches. With this in mind, before any analysis of its reception, it becomes important to understand the narrative of *Lucky, the Hero!*.

Lucky, the Hero! Synopsis

Scene I: *Big Problems at No Problems Farm*

The narrator communicates directly with the audience, introducing the fictional No Problems Farm and the community's reluctance to talk about HIV. He explains that he is going to tell them a story about a young man named Lucky, and how his experiences changed the community for the better. This scene introduces the issue of HIV/AIDS stigma and discrimination, highlighting a prevailing reluctance in the community to discuss sensitive topics such as sex, condoms, or AIDS.

Scene II: *A Real Ladies' Man*

The audience learns from the narrator that Lucky has had many sexual relationships. He dances with Nita, a socially popular young woman, to the Afrikaans pop song "Losplappie" (translated to mean "loose rag," itself a reference to casual sexual encounters). The narrator reminds the audience that HIV does not discriminate on the basis of age, race, gender, or sexuality. Lucky is rejected by the young woman for refusing to agree to use a condom. Later, after hearing a radio show about HIV awareness, Lucky realizes that he has put his health and the health of others at risk by not practicing safe sex. The scene presents the risks associated with unsafe sex with multiple partners.

Scene III: *HIV-Positive*

Lucky goes to his local clinic to take an HIV test where he learns that he is HIV-positive. He receives information on his condition from Theresa, the local nurse, who simultaneously provides information to the audience about ARV medications and maintaining one's health while living with HIV. She informs him that if he stops drinking heavily, smoking "dagga" (cannabis), and takes the correct medication, then he could live a long and happy life.

Scene IV: *Maybe You Infected Me!*

After listening to another radio broadcast discussing HIV disclosure, Lucky decides to confide in his smooth-talking and long-standing best friend Two-Time Tokie. Tokie dances provocatively into the scene wearing dark sunglasses to a rendition of Right Said Fred's "Too Sexy." Walking into the audience, he engages with those in the front rows, flirting and playfully soliciting a number of individuals, before turning to face his friend. After multiple reassurances from Tokie that nothing could change their friendship, Lucky discloses his HIV status. Tokie initially dismisses it as a joke but then rejects Lucky's friendship due to his ignorance of the virus and its transmission, upon realizing that Lucky is not joking. The scene provides health-related information about HIV transmission and thematically acknowledges the risks associated with HIV status disclosure due to AIDS-related stigma.

Scene V: *Just Be Strong*

The audience learns that the entire No Problems Farm community has abandoned Lucky because of his HIV status. Lucky visits his local clinic again and is comforted by Theresa, who explains that ignorance is the cause of the community's response to him. He later calls the radio program from Scene II. He talks to DJ Chenin Blanc to ask for her advice on how to cope with his situation and explains that the community has been fabricating defamatory stories about him. DJ Chenin Blanc reassures him that by knowing his status, he is showing that he respects himself and others. Lucky decides to take matters into his own hands and be positive about his situation. He exclaims that he has a plan of action before running offstage.

Scene VI: *Protection*!?

The scene opens with Tokie dancing in a club with Nita. Tokie seduces her and they agree to leave the club together. When she mentions that they must use protection, however, Tokie gets angry and says that real men do not use condoms. Seeing his offense, Nita retracts her condition that they must use protection and remarks that condoms are not necessary. At this point, an unknown figure dressed in red overalls appears and begins to sing about protecting oneself and getting tested for HIV to the melody of Frankie Valli's "Can't Take My Eyes Off You." He then hands condoms to both Tokie and Nita. Condom use, sugar daddies, and pressure to engage in unsafe sex are explored in this scene.

Scene VII: *HIV in the Blood and Seeing Other Women*

DJ Chenin Blanc opens the scene with more information on HIV transmission. She commends a young man who has been spotted all around No Problems Farm, wearing red overalls and handing out condoms. She dubs him Capt. AIDS-fighter. The scene shifts to Tokie, who is about to be physically intimate with Nita. When Tokie's pregnant wife Theresa returns home from her shift at the local clinic, however, Tokie tries to cover up the situation with little effect. Exasperated with the situation, Nita reveals herself and they begin to verbally fight. At this point, Capt. AIDS-fighter appears and tells Tokie that his reckless sexual behavior could risk infecting his wife and unborn child with HIV and that real men think of their families first, not their sexual desires for other women. The group then continues to sing about condom use to the tune of "Can't Take My Eyes Off You." The central theme of the scene is to remain faithful to a romantic partner.

Scene VIII: *Your Future Is Your Choice*!

The scene opens with Tokie expressing his disapproval that everyone is talking about HIV and condoms since Capt. AIDS-fighter appeared in the community. He angrily states that he does not feel like a man anymore. The community, however, think differently. Theresa and DJ Chenin Blanc berate Tokie for not getting tested, not using condoms, and his terrible treatment of Lucky when he disclosed his HIV status. Tokie realizes his mistakes and wonders how to make this up to his best friend. In this moment, Capt. AIDS-fighter appears and reveals his identity. Tokie apologizes and Lucky accepts, saying that it is in the past and they all need to move forward. The narrator explains to the audience how a positive attitude can change your own life and the lives of those around you. The scene ends with a reimagined rendition of Gloria Gaynor's "I Will Survive," with the lyrics altered to reflect the message of acceptance toward PLHIV. The actors mingle with the audience members throughout the musical number, encouraging them to dance, and become involved in the energetic finale.

Musical Effervescence in the *Lucky, the Hero!* Finale

The rural Free State school hall is filled with high school students, their crisp school uniforms sending a vivid splash of cobalt blue across the entire breadth of the space. The performance at this remote area near the border with Lesotho began about an hour ago. Teachers stand at uneven intervals around where the students are sitting, presumably to maintain discipline, but they need not do so. Each of the students has been transfixed by the unfolding narrative of *Lucky, the Hero!* pulled into the performance—mostly figuratively but at times quite literally—by the interactive and participatory elements of the show and the unfettered charisma of its actors. At this end stage of the performance, the audience has been primed by sixty minutes of narrative, character development, role modeling, comedy, musical interludes, and dramatic intrigue. Through these elements, a connection to the purpose of HIV prevention is established within the minds of the audience, solidifying the first step toward musical effervescence.

Each member of the cast is standing on the stage, facing the audience as they begin to sing, visually signaling the impending final musical number. In stark contrast to most of the performances that preceded it, the opening to the climactic finale begins with unassuming serenity. Each actor individually sings a melodic line one at a time. The vocals are tranquil, sung in free time over a subtle harmony created by a smooth synthesized backing track.

> Narrator: So that is our story, it has come to an end.
> Theresa: So please try to remember and tell a friend.
> Nita: About positive Lucky's . . .
> DJ Chenin Blanc: Positive way.
> All (in unison): He's no different than anyone here today.
>
> (Personal recording of the *Lucky, the Hero!* finale, 2014)

As the actors sing the end of their individual lines that set up the grand finale, it is clear that the participants can sense the anticipation. The cast sings the concluding line of the opening melodies in unison. The final cadential pitch is held, suspended by the singers to build a sense of anticipation, the kind of psycho-sonic tension of withholding the harmonic resolution from dominant to tonic. The audience begins shouting and hollering in support, while others hoot in excitement as the dominant harmony hangs in the air. Embodied potential energy begins to manifest into physical actions. Participants shift in their seats while others clap in anticipation.

A thumping kick drum and snare rhythm finally breaks the anticipation for the musical finale. The dominant harmonic tension is released into tonic resolution, and the explosive entrance of the uplifting chorus to "I Will Survive" bursts from the theater company's PA speakers, providing the main impetus for collective synchronicity and the sonic structuring of bodies. The moment the main musical theme begins, a group of participants jumps up from their seats and starts dancing and shouting; the second step toward musical effervescence is now in motion. The actors smile broadly as they perform a synchronized dance routine, clapping on the main beats of each bar and inviting the audience to do the same. The positive sounds of "I Will Survive" flow from the group's speakers as the song is now in full swing, with all the actors singing fully harmonized melodic lines with lyrics of tolerance and hope for an HIV-free generation over a full backing track.

> No Problems people, learnt their lessons today,
> To reject someone positive is not the way
> So why don't you go and get a test, put your mind at rest
> It's better to know your state, so you can choose your own fate
>
> (Personal recording of the *Lucky, the Hero!* finale, 2014)

The music and choreography emphasize each beat immediately after the words "I will survive" throughout the chorus with digital trumpet staccato chords. The word "survive" lands on the first beat of each bar, followed by the accented staccatos on beat two. The actors dance in choreographed steps from side to side, throwing their hands out to meet each staccato trumpet blast with abounding energy. Without the need to verbalize it, the musical number loudly proclaims itself to be the final musical outro to the whole performance, and the participants are eager to join in. By this time, half of the hall is already on their feet, while others pull their friends up out of their seats. The third step toward musical effervescence begins to coalesce as patches of sporadic synchronicity settle into wider-spread collective entrainment of bodies.

> Everyone is affected
> If someone's infected, don't have them rejected,
> So listen up, oh listen up
> If we all stick together, we can conquer HIV
> And in a few short years, we'll be free.
>
> (Personal recording of the *Lucky, the Hero!* finale, 2014)

While beginning with only a small number of highly animated participants, a high-intensity, affectively charged atmosphere has engulfed the hall as the theater group's grand musical finale reflects and reverberates from every wall and window. In real-time, this process has taken only a matter of seconds, but that is all the time that is needed before the hall erupts into a musically driven effervescent assembly with heightened affective states of being together with others in the music. The sound of the participants' vocalizations begins to entrain with the pulse of "I Will Survive," quickly developing into syncopated "wooh" articulations on beats two and four, with many others clapping their hands. As I pan my camera across the audience, I witness Durkheim's electricity reaching its voltaic tendrils to the back of the hall as people begin jumping up onto benches and chairs (indeed, sometimes onto each other) or climbing up the equipment stacked against the walls. Others still swing their hats and scarves in the air above their heads and cheer. The exclamations from the learners grow so loud that they begin to overpower the theater group's PA system. Not even the teachers are immune to the intoxicating effervescence, as they clap their hands and swing their hips to the resounding anthem. The wave of effervescence flows through the crowd, with animation leaping from person to person, Durkheim's electricity flowing from conduit to conduit. I watch through my camera lens as participants release the energy that has built up over the course of the performance, with no explicit prompting from the theater group. They jump to their feet and move their bodies with increasing vigor to the music industry standard 4/4 pulse, with broad smiles on their faces as they lose themselves in the musicking experience, entrained in musical effervescence.

> We will survive, we will survive
> As long as we know how to live, we know we'll stay alive
> We will survive, we will survive

As long as we know how to love, we know we'll stay alive
Because HIV and AIDS is everybody's fight
We will survive!

(Personal recording of the *Lucky, the Hero!* finale, 2014)

The students move further from their seats, spreading out among the empty spaces of the hall, using more of the performance space to express themselves. Some sit down once again but continue to dance in their seats, while others remain on their feet, clapping, chanting, whistling, shouting, throwing their hands above their heads, and anticipating the staccato trumpet punctuations between the theater group's lyrics. Almost as soon as the display has begun, the song is over, but a heightened emotional state has been created. Rasping trumpets accentuate the rhythm of the final melody, which carries the powerful final lyrical declaration, "We will survive!" The one-minute musical number that the narrative has been building to has transformed the assembly hall. Socially prescribed boundaries and hierarchical etiquette have been temporarily dissolved as the relationships between performers, listeners, students, and teachers are reshaped and reimagined within participatory musicking.

The students take their seats again shortly after the music has stopped but they are not settled. A familiar amplified voice resonates throughout the hall as Florance, the group's administrator, capitalizes on the room's energy: "Give it up for *Lucky, the Hero!*" The audience claps their hands and screams emphatically. "Did you enjoy that!?" he shouts into his microphone as he takes to the stage to rapturous applause and screams. "Did you *enjoy* that!?" he exclaims once again, further building upon the participants' energy. With each question, the screaming becomes louder and the flailing arms of the participants more jubilant. It is at this point, with the hall electrified with musical effervescence and all eyes fixed on Florance, that he invites the participants to take an HIV test and know their status. Hundreds rush to the temporary testing facilities set up toward a small collection of rooms adjacent to the main performance space. Within a few minutes, a queue has formed through the hall, out the door, and around the building. The work is slow and the demand high, but within an hour or so, the overwhelming majority of participants leave the performance space knowing their HIV status. Performances such as this provide potent examples of musical effervescence and its application within an HIV testing drive. The energy of hundreds of people entrained through rhythm and pulse, collectively focused, and affectively energized through a collective musicking experience is channeled into a positive health outcome.

Just as Durkheim described collectives that appeared to transcend the world in front of them for an imagined reality of possibilities, so too have I witnessed such scenes in the performance spaces of the *Lucky, the Hero!* shows. The kinds of manic creativity outlined in Chapter 3 seem to nourish the minds of the participants with belief and possibility. Where Durkheim posited the formulation of ideal worlds in the thoughts of those in the grip of collective effervescence through the presence and proximity of bodies and minds, my observations have found similar, albeit more modest expressions. Durkheim's manic creativity manifests within this health promotion environment as a strengthening of self-efficacy. First outlined by behavioral psychologist Albert Bandura (1994) through his formulation of social cognitive theory, self-efficacy describes a belief that one's actions can lead to achievable results and has come to form a crucial component of contemporary public health promotion initiatives.

As participants who have used the on-site testing facilities begin to make their way home, I take the opportunity to see if anyone is willing to chat about their perceptions and experiences during the performance. As I mingle among the crowd, a small group is in the process of creating a beautiful rendition of the final musical number "I Will Survive" in rich, multipart harmony. Waiting until their reimagined a cappella rendition had concluded, I introduce myself to who I would come to know as Sesi, Palesa, Mpho, and Bongi.[1] When I asked them to describe how they are feeling now that the show had finished, their responses highlighted the emotional impact that *Lucky, the Hero!* made.

Sesi: I feel great and wonderful. We feel like we can do anything now, right?
Palesa: Yes!
Bongi: Yeah!
Sesi: There's always so much bad news about life, but right now, we can do anything we set our hearts on. God has filled my heart with love.
Palesa: Preach, my sister! God is hearing you.
Sesi: There are so many problems here but AIDS doesn't have to be one of them. We have the power to change our future and we can do it, just like the people in the play said: we will survive.

(Interview with *Lucky, the Hero!* participants, August 2014)

Sesi begins to sing part of the tune from the theater group's finale. The other girls clap along and switch between dancing together while adding beautifully intricate harmonies and laughing among themselves.

Sesi: Lord, we have love and music here! Music is the sound of God in all of us.
Mpho: God gave us the gift of singing. We Africans, we sing because it is in our souls. Those people [the ETC], they have soul. You can hear it in their songs.
Sesi: We are all together, we have to free ourselves from the virus, from the fear and the hate. The message is important and these singers, the ones in the performance, they have God in their hearts, they are warriors for God.

(Interview with *Lucky, the Hero!* participants, August 2014)

The process of manic creativity through which new social realities and relationships may be conceptualized can be a profound and quasi-spiritual experience. Indeed, Durkheim's own conceptualization of collective effervescence resulted from his observation of rituals that exhibited intense spiritual associations, as outlined in *The Elementary Forms of the Religious Life* ([1912] 2008). That music and song are associated with the divine is hardly new; communal singing has long been a way for many South African cultures to express their faith in the divine and strengthen community bonds through ritual. A number of these practices were then incorporated into the syncretic Christian faiths that developed as a result of European settler colonialism, highlighted in Chapter 4. But what is of note here is the transcendental states of being cultivated among the participants in an event with no association to religion and makes no overt reference to God or spirituality. While the overwhelming majority of South Africans identify as Christian, *Lucky, the Hero!* is a secular performance. For these participants, their experiences were divine, the message righteous, and the vessels "warriors for God." The kinds of manic creativity that manifest in a euphoric self-efficacy are buoyed by their associations with a higher purpose. As Durkheim noted, effervescence lifts participants beyond that which could be expected in everyday life, and in doing so, the effects of musical effervescence may take on spiritual significance according to the heights that one finds oneself.

The events described above illustrate that *Lucky, the Hero!* has the potential to elicit surging emotional and kinetic responses from audience members. The most immediate results of these experiences can be found within the number of individuals who utilize the testing facilities provided by @Heart. Less easily quantifiable effects, however, can be observed within the behaviors of the participants after the shows, which will be discussed in some detail in the following section. Many of the participants, uplifted by their experience of musical effervescence, leave the performance space with a positive frame of mind, renewed belief in the possibility of an HIV-free generation, and knowing their HIV status.

Sustaining Effervescent Assemblies: Structuring Post-Show Transitions Toward Health Outcomes

The intense emotional surges associated with the musical effervescence cultivated by the *Lucky, the Hero!* performances, while transient in nature (as all emotions are), often continued beyond the temporal and spatial boundaries of the original performance. Those who participated—the effervescent assemblies—were often reluctant to come down from their electrically charged heightened emotional states. When I next accompanied the theater group on an intervention, this phenomenon became strikingly apparent to me during the second performance at a state school in rural Mpumalanga province.

In a large agricultural facility in Mpumalanga, a few miles from the town of Ermelo, the theater group has just finished its performance, and the atmosphere is energetic and animated. As is customary after the shows, the group's sound technician begins to play pop club beats through the speakers while the focus of the intervention shifts to the voluntary HIV testing drive. We begin to load some of the equipment back into the van. Within a few minutes, a small group begins to dance to the music. The technician responds by raising the volume to emphasize the thumping bass pulse. As he does so, one of the more extroverted participants jumps in front of the mixing desk and proceeds to dance proficiently.

Within moments, the small crowd begins to grow as others are drawn to the scene. They congregate around him and cheer him on with loud whistles and yells. A group of individuals who had been making their way away from the facility turn around and come back to join the large circle that is forming around the dancers. Some of the more confident participants show off their dance moves and physical prowess in the newly created performance space in front of the mixing desk. A young man in a blue sweater makes his way into the circle with staccato movements to the pulse of the club rhythms. Fluid synthesized notes bounce from pitch to pitch, emphasizing harmonically important frequencies over the driving bass beat. The sound of a distorted marimba provides a countermelody to the smooth harmonic tones. Once inside the dance circle, with all eyes on him, the young man in the blue sweater skillfully jumps from one foot to the other, sliding his feet along the ground beneath him as he does so.

The crowd has now doubled in size, with a small performance area in front of the mixing desk being the only free space left. As the song ends, it is replaced with another equally infectious dance beat. The dancer in the blue sweater retreats from the circle and is supplanted by another, eagerly waiting for a moment in the spotlight. Pop club music continues to thump from the speakers as the circle of musicking participants cheer on their peers. Some enter the circle in pairs, stepping in time to the beat as they do so, then manically, yet dexterously, throw their bodies into impressive maneuvers and momentary poses, while others clap and hoot from the sidelines. The creative expression and movement of people between the dance circle and @Heart's testing area continue until all the equipment has been packed away, except the PA system and the mixing desk. Finally, when there is nothing more to pack into the theater group's van and the spectacle has stretched the intervention over its allotted time, the signal is given to fade out the music. As quickly as the circle had formed to the sound of the pop club beats, so too does it disappear.

While not officially part of the show, the theater group implicitly recognizes that cultivating an additional musicking event maintains the energy of the performance throughout the HIV testing period. While it does not always culminate in such a display, my observations suggest that the music helps to facilitate the transition from the high-energy performance to the testing drive. What is noteworthy about this particular situation is the manner in which this scene unfolded, and the ease with which it did so. Without a word to one another on the subject, or any formal oversight, this group of participants were able to arrange themselves in a highly organized fashion: they selected a suitable area as their performance space; others, though eager to have a good view of the spectacle, instinctively knew to give the area in front of the mixing desk a wide berth; and the flow of dancers in and out of the performance space was smooth and organized, with no two dancers unwittingly sharing the floor at the same time or interrupting the groove of another.

The dance circle is indicative of musicking's capacity for the spatial and temporal structuring of large groups. Given that music is able to structure inchoate bodies into shared space and time (DeNora 2013), it provides a useful tool that may be employed by the theater group in an effort to sonically scaffold the transitional space and time between the main performance and the following HIV testing drive. While the coordinators could use more traditional methods of directing participants to the testing areas, and often do, the strength of employing musicking to support the transition from performance to testing is that it helps the theater group to regulate the space without explicitly telling people what to do. The group must be mindful that their encouragement toward a particular behavior is not misinterpreted as pressure that may elicit resistance from the participants in the manner of the old Confucian adage noted earlier in Chapter 5.

To elaborate on this point, the concept of reactance in social psychology suggests that direct instructions from a place of perceived authority may quite easily be interpreted as an infringement of personal freedom (Brehm 1966). Reactance is described as "an unpleasant motivational arousal that emerges when people experience a threat to or loss of their free behaviors" (Steindl et al. 2015, 205). Such perceived threats to personal freedom often arise from impersonal situational factors (Clee and Wicklund 1980; Brehm and Brehm 1981), thus emphasizing the importance of cultivating connections between both health information providers and the participants on the one hand, and between the participants themselves on the other. A state of reactance is characterized by behavioral and cognitive efforts to re-establish personal agency and freedom of decision-making through hostility to suggested instructions (Steindl et al. 2015). While the theater group uses musicking as a counterbalance to reactance throughout the show, it is employed particularly impactfully during these key transitional periods in which participants are informed of the available testing facilities.

One of the main strengths of using songs and musical experiences to combat reactance is its ubiquity and the normalcy of music to provide structure to various activities of our everyday lives (DeNora 2000). While the musicking event displayed high levels of embodied energy, the phenomenon was remarkably unremarkable. This spontaneous musicking experience, while energetic and animated, dissipated as soon as the music faded, illustrating another of a potentially indefinite number of often overlooked applied musicking methodologies hidden in plain sight (Walker 2024).

The theater group's use of songs to maintain the energy of the performance into the HIV testing drive that follows demonstrates an understanding that music is able to maintain enhanced energetic states of musical effervescence among participants. While the duration and intensity of these experiences varied between performances, its use provided an entertaining reason to remain in the vicinity of the testing site long after the main performance had ended, heightening the probability of utilizing the facilities. Moreover, the animated dancing is a symptom of the emotive and highly connective experience, an affective overflow from the performance structured into coherence through "mutually tuning-in," to borrow the term from Alfred Schütz (1951).[2] It illustrates a potent example of embodied sensorial and emotional expression and coordination of thought and action through rhythm and pulse.

Hearing with the Body: Embodiment of Music in Effervescent Assemblies

One of the arguments made in this book is that musical experiences, and songs in particular, can be important, yet often overlooked, components in creating effervescent assemblies. The power of such assemblies has frequently been harnessed for social and health outcomes within the South African AIDS crisis. Within the natural and medical sciences, it is standard practice to test a hypothesis using a control group, that is to say, a neutral set of participants or data against which one can compare the results of an experiment. Opportunities to implement such a model within ethnomusicological or anthropological research, with their focus on the "messiness of the experiential" (Ahmed 2010, 22), are extremely rare.

While accompanying a theater group that performs the same show to a number of similar audiences in a short space of time largely prevents the use of ethnography within the communities who are participating in the performances, a silver lining of this situation is that I was able to observe how different collections of participants responded to the show. On one particular occasion, during a performance at a rural high school, I stumbled quite by chance upon a situation that demonstrates the importance of the songs within the *Lucky, the Hero!* show to cultivate the effervescent assemblies. What a scholar of the natural sciences might refer to as controlling for all other variables except the music, I witnessed only one performance in the time I spent with the Educational Theatre Company that failed to cultivate the kind of effervescent assembly described earlier in this chapter, and this was it.

Traveling through the vast expanses of grazing pastures and maize fields, the high summer sun beats through every window of the small minibus that I am sharing with the Educational Theatre Company. Gently tapping the driver on the shoulder, I am told that we are somewhere in rural Free State Province between Ficksburg and Hlohlolwane. I return to my seat and gaze out at the villagers and small hamlets that glide by the window every now and then. The bus is quiet. A very early morning flight from Cape Town to Bloemfontein has rendered the usually animated and raucous character of the minivan road trip relatively subdued.

By late morning, the paved roads have disappeared, promptly awakening any of the actors who may have dozed off during the journey. Sunbaked and dusty gravel roads lead us to tall and rusty iron gates that stand open and appear to have stopped working long ago. Passing an ominous sign announcing in three different languages (isiZulu, English, and Afrikaans) an extensive list of prohibited items, clothing, and behavior, awkwardly juxtaposed with a large sign missing flakes of peeled paint welcoming us to the high school, the minibus proceeds into the school grounds.

Upon arriving at our destination, the theater group and I learn that the area is currently experiencing a blackout due to "load shedding." This is a policy of state-sanctioned, intentionally implemented rolling blackouts to reduce the burden on the national energy grid. No power would ultimately result in a largely unamplified version of the performance. As men in blue overalls finish setting out plastic chairs under a large, stained tarpaulin marquee, the issue of amplification is partially resolved by the sound technician's fast thinking. As the rest of the group continues to set up, he parks the group's minivan as close to the tent as possible in the hope that the van's sound system could act as a replacement for the PA system, playing the music through its speakers. Children begin to flow into the performance space and take their seats. The hum of muted conversations grows as the participants continue to fill the marquee until it is bustling with the noise of hundreds of chatting school children.

Until this moment, the process seems identical to every other show that has been performed at a high school. Since performances such as this are relatively uncommon for these remote schools, the students are excited to see the show. However, as the opening musical number struggles to be heard from the van's speakers, it is immediately clear that this performance will be very different from the others. The theater group tries valiantly to engage the attention of the audience while striving to project their unamplified voices. The poor acoustics of the tent and the increasing hum of hundreds of school children muttering among themselves make this an unenviable task. Participants at the back, who despite the efforts of the performers cannot hear the dialogues or songs, quickly lose interest and begin entertaining themselves in other ways. Some look at their phones, while others initiate group conversations with those sitting around them. Florance, the Educational Theatre Company's administrator, flashes a concerned glance at one of the teachers. With an expression of displeasure, he gestures his head toward the audience. The hum has grown so loud and distracting for the actors that they are beginning to look uncomfortable. Taking note of the situation, the performance is stopped and the children are given an ultimatum by the school staff: either sit quietly or go back to class.

The narrative is able to continue its journey toward its ultimate conclusion, but there is little enthusiasm from the audience as the singers begin to build toward the finale.

> Narrator: So that is our story, it has come to an end.
> Theresa: So please try to remember and tell a friend.
> Nita: About positive Lucky's . . .
> DJ Chenin Blanc: Positive way.
> All (in unison): He's no different than anyone here today.
>
> (Personal recording of the *Lucky, the Hero!* finale, 2014)

The familiar melodies are faint and powerless as they attempt in vain to build toward the finale. As the musical number reaches what would normally be its climactic finale, the learners remain relatively motionless and simply observe the proceedings. Noticing that something is wrong, Florance intervenes in an attempt to involve the audience. "Clap your hands, everyone!" he calls into the crowd. The neutered sounds of "I Will Survive" labor to fill the performance space as Ricardo, who plays the lead role of Lucky, begins to gyrate and jump up and down on the spot, desperately trying to maintain the attention of the audience. "Clap your hands!" Florance shouts again, raising his hands above his head and clapping his hands together in wide arcs.

The rest of the theater group start clapping along in encouragement, and gradually some members of the audience begin to participate. Some of the learners begin to shout and hoot and whistle from the back of the tent, as the clapped beat and participation seem to thaw what was previously an unengaged crowd. Most, however, despite clapping and smiling, remain composed. As the theater group strike their poses for the final "We will survive!" the notes ring out into a sea of staring faces who are no longer able to clap along. A second or two of uncomfortable silence passes before Florance is once again forced to intervene. "Give a round of applause for *Lucky, the Hero!*" he yells into the crowd. The learners dutifully applaud the performance. Florance then begins his usual post-performance discussion with the audience, shouting "did you enjoy that?" A rather lackluster "yes" emanates from the learners before he playfully demands:

"did you enjoy that!?" "Yes!" replied the children. This time, the response is slightly more enthusiastic in tone and volume. Florance once again encourages the participants to know their status but with such little enthusiasm, only a handful of learners utilize the facilities. In stark contrast with the impromptu dance circle noted earlier, the testing drive is over before we have even finished loading the equipment back into the van.

The differences between this performance and the others that I observed were stark. The previous day, the theater group had performed the same show to a different school in a nearby area without any interruption in the electricity supply. For all intents and purposes, the participants in each of those two performances were extremely similar. They were both school performances of roughly the same size, age, and gender composition, from similar socioeconomic backgrounds, cultures, and geographic areas. Both audiences participated in the same show with the same actors, essentially controlling for all other variables. The only denominator that was missing between them was the lack of high-impact musical accompaniment during the second show.

This unamplified performance highlights something that, thus far, this book has not addressed: that sounds—and subsequently music—may be inhibited in a variety of ways. While music has been shown throughout this book to be a remarkably powerful force, it is not an unbounded one (Tausig 2019). That is to say, the sonorous qualities of musicking and the auralities discussed in this book are not limitless in their physical expressions. Barriers may be erected to dampen unwelcome sounds, music may be psychologically tuned out, rows of buildings may block the noise from a protest (as was the case while walking through Greenmarket Square in the opening ethnography of this book), or the physiological capabilities of the human vocal apparatus may be insufficient to resonate through large performance spaces.

Space is an important component of atmosphere, and in turn, affects atmospheres and effervescence. The "feel" of a room or an area is often readily interpreted by those who are within it. As Jack (2021) notes, the "sensorial aspects of human experience influence the interpretation of scenarios and potentialities of action" (501). Of course, atmosphere is not inherently bound to space, but it does permeate it, and the transformative properties of music significantly influence the perception of space and the actions one may take within it (Fischer-Lichte 2007).

While music was present in a muted and limited way, it was not felt. The thumping bass of the pop music that I could usually feel in my chest from the theater group's PA system was conspicuously absent. For Schneck and Berger (2006), "music impacts the entire human organism, from the individual atoms, molecules, and cells to the most complex tissues, organs, and systems" (92). Since our entire body interprets acoustic vibrations, rather than just our auditory sensory apparatus, the conscious mind is not fully aware of the extent of the body's response sometimes until long after the event (Schneck and Berger 2006). In essence then, the physiological responses to stimuli that occur with limited cognitive input are part of a more holistic sensorial experience. Amplification, therefore, becomes an important tool to engender participation within hybrid presentational/participatory performances such as *Lucky, the Hero!*, the sonic interconnectedness afforded by its space-filling properties and temporal structuring of bodies reinforces the organic participation threaded throughout the performance. This is, of course, not to say that musical effervescence cannot occur without thumping amplified music, but rather that in some form or other, music must be both embodied physically as well as registered psychologically (Friedson 1996), it must be felt as well as heard.

Conclusion

The *Lucky, the Hero!* performances provide powerful examples of musical effervescence in action. The participants are exposed to an emotionally charged theater and musicking event in the form of a short but high-energy performance. Throughout the hour-long show, participants are vicariously led through a variety of emotive situations from boisterous and uplifting to sympathetic and moving. If delivered successfully, the performance is able to energize participants considerably, largely through a contagious emotional and affective response that spreads from participant to participant. This response is embodied, expressed, and communicated in abstract and physical ways, but barely registered as out of the ordinary and certainly not clearly defined (Wetherell 2012). In this way, *Lucky, the Hero!* employs both cognitive and affective multi-sensorial communication to present health information to participants.

The tactical use of participation builds upon the show's narrative to develop connections, as members of the audience are drawn in to become part of the show through dialogues and musical numbers. By the final scenes, affective responses are displayed among a progressively entrained collective, as individuals experience increasing spatial interconnectedness and temporal synchronicity. Affective experiences are shared among the audience as the effervescent assembly develops, usually from a small number of highly animated participants. As the sonorous and harmonic tensions are built, there is a visceral sense of Durkheim's electricity among the participants. The musical finale, with its upbeat tempo, uplifting lyrics, driving beat, and inviting choreography, provides the final catalyst for musical effervescence. Explosive kinetic and emotional energy is released within the minute-long finale through dancing, shouting, waving, clapping, and other intense displays of musically entrained collective effervescence.

Contemporary theories of crowd behavior, musical experiences, and social psychology, when considered alone, are unable to adequately account for the high-energy displays and manic creativity cultivated by the *Lucky, the Hero!* shows. The participatory musical and musicking performances entrain large numbers of individuals in musical effervescence through embodied sensorial experience, rhythm, pulse, and the combined and self-perpetuating electricity of assembling with others. Indeed, I have not been immune to this phenomenon either. Even as someone who has observed the *Lucky, the Hero!* performances many times, who has watched the group rehearse and perform, who has read the script, spoken with those who created it, socialized with the actors, analyzed the music, and developed an in-depth understanding of the rationale, methods, and health and social outcomes that *Lucky, the Hero!* strives to achieve, I am still influenced by the affective wave of effervescent electricity created by the performances.

With the difficulties experienced throughout the performance during the rolling blackouts, it became clear that the sonorous vibrations must be felt in a visceral and embodied way; otherwise, the technique fails. The success of creating musical effervescence is dependent on the culmination of a number of factors, including purpose, participation, synchronicity and entrainment, and the embodiment of the musicking experience (Walker 2022c). By utilizing the sonorous and rhythmic qualities of music, the actors are able to cultivate heightened affective and emotional states of interconnectedness, euphoria, and manic creativity among the audience. Bodies and minds entrained in musical effervescence become open to new social realities, ideas, and behaviors. Susceptibility to new ways of being remains powerful and influential for some time after the effervescent event. While long-term solutions must involve ongoing support and access to community-level health services, musical effervescence is effectively harnessed by the Educational Theatre Company to persuade participants to utilize the on-site HIV testing facilities and know their HIV status.

It should be clear from the case studies discussed thus far in this book that live participatory performance can be fertile ground for the cultivation of musical effervescence. However, issues related to amplification noted in this chapter raise interesting questions regarding the use of audio technologies and their place within health interventions. Moreover, as I have noted in the discussion of Band Aid in Chapter 4 since the 1980s audiovisual media have carved out a significant space within humanitarianism and public health campaigning across the world. The ubiquity of audiovisual mass media approaches cannot be ignored within this book's exploration of the songs of the South African AIDS crisis. The following chapter is dedicated to examining such themes.

Notes

1 Each of the names has been changed to protect the identities of the participants.

2 Alfred Schütz described the fundamentally social nature of music as defined by what he termed the "mutual tuning-in relationships" in his article "Making Music Together" (1951). His observation that music helped to engender nonverbal social relationships between people was one of the earliest incarnations of phenomena that ethnomusicologists would likely now describe using terms like "musicking" and "entrainment."

9

Music Videos as Mass-Media HIV/AIDS Awareness and Prevention

The capacity of music to enhance emotive shared experiences is widely regarded as one of its most important qualities (Hesmondhalgh 2013). Understanding the social aspects of music has been a defining feature of ethnomusicological inquiry. The discipline has prioritized the analysis of musical culture through situated experiential data. This has yielded significant insight into lived experiences, but a holistic approach to understanding the influence of musical experiences, particularly as they relate to health and social outcomes, must also include discussions of the effects that recorded music has on the lives of billions of individuals across the world every day. While the social aspects of music are primarily demonstrated by its most participatory forms, it would be an oversight not to examine the application of recorded music within South Africa's HIV/AIDS epidemic.

Turino (2008) outlines a spectrum of musical activity through which we may determine the participatory properties of various aspects of musicking. He notes that what he refers to as *participatory* and *presentational* performances occupy the more interactive end of the continuum, with what he refers to as *high-fidelity recordings* and *studio audio art* residing at the opposite end (90–1). While each plot on this spectrum can be considered a form of musicking, it serves to demonstrate the broad range of musicking activities from live participatory events to recorded music and illustrates that the most presentational or pre-recorded examples of musicking activities still exercise significant, if transitory, influence on human life. Even the postindustrial global north, with its consumer cultures and commodified popular musics, is subject to the collective ordering of social life through music. As one music sociologist puts it, musicking involving recorded music is still able to "structure the happening" of our everyday lives (DeNora 2000, 113).

Moving on from the well-trodden ground of participatory music, it is important that audiovisual media is not ignored. The vast majority of our social interactions do not fall toward the immediately participatory and presentational end of Turino's spectrum, but this small selection of musicking garners the vast majority of scholarly attention. One could quite easily argue, as Crossley (2020) does, that because high-fidelity recordings may engender equally participatory and socially connective behavior they deserve equal scholarly attention. The symbolic and material properties of music's sonorous qualities are used on a daily basis to create spaces for different social functions. Music is used to structure relaxed intimacy in restaurants or embodied rhythm and pulse in nightclubs. Indeed, a fascinating observation of Blacking's (1974) often-discussed definition of music as "humanly organised sound" is the additional propensity of music to sonorously (soundly?) organize humans.

This organization of individuals and actions can be found throughout our daily lives and often manifests through the behaviors and social conventions associated with various types of music. DeNora highlights this property of music in her first monograph, *Music in Everyday Life* (2000), specifically discussing the ways in which music can be applied, perhaps unconsciously, toward organizing otherwise disconnected individuals such that their actions appear to be mutually oriented and coordinated. While the multitude of musical experiences we encounter day to day are often not consciously perceived, these experiences nevertheless play an enormous role in how we live our lives. They help us to make conscious and unconscious assessments about social situations based on previous experience, associations with signs and symbols, and the kinds of atmospheric environments such music may cultivate. Less immediate than the more participatory forms of musicking, these (usually recorded) forms of musical experience are no less impactful on human life and provide opportunities, even in the most consumerist of contexts, to guide human experience in various spaces.

Moreover, few things can alter the atmosphere of a given social situation like music. Its space-filling properties are useful in creating ambience that subconsciously influences behavior. As has been discussed in Chapter 5, much scholarship has discussed the profound influence of music in the commercial sphere (Taylor 2012, 2016; Elmashhara and Soares 2020) as well as its potential to improve athletic performance during exercise (Terry et al. 2020). Likewise, Blacking (1987) himself observed that music was simultaneously able to engender "unique ways of feeling" (40) within individuals as well as "waves of feelings" (76) between them.

In the digital age of social media and viral content, the music video or small sound bite has reaffirmed its position in online popular culture across the world. I have already discussed in Chapter 5 how and why what I have termed the "Band Aid" method of health and humanitarian campaigning can be highly successful in fundraising, but this chapter looks more closely at this approach within the South African AIDS epidemic for awareness and prevention. While there are many potential anthems to discuss, the focus of analysis in this chapter is "ZAZI," a song and music video developed by Johns Hopkins University, the production company Joe Public, and the South African National AIDS Council (SANAC) as part of a women's sexual and reproductive health campaign of the same name. ZAZI was launched in 2013 to catalyze a national discussion on gender inequality, female reproductive health, and HIV/AIDS. During my interview with the deputy director of the ZAZI campaign in Cape Town, Bronwyn Pierce, she elaborated on the objectives of the campaign, suggesting that ZAZI was a vehicle for creating a social movement around women's issues.

> Primarily we want to deal with issues around HIV and AIDS, as well as teenage pregnancy, and all the other sexual and reproductive health issues that we know young women are facing in South Africa. (Interview with Bronwyn Pierce, February 2014)

The song features South African soul singer Zonke Dikana and Johannesburg-based poet King Nova. As a national campaign associated with South African performing artists, the "ZAZI" music video presents an opportunity to examine the application of audiovisual media for health and social outcomes relating to the HIV/AIDS epidemic. Before any empirical data may be fruitfully explored, it is important to contextualize such data through analysis of the song and its accompanying music video.

The "ZAZI" Music Video

There is no definitive approach to interpreting music, but it is reasonable to suggest—as many musicologists and ethnomusicologists do—that we may understand some of the potential meanings associated with music through hermeneutic analysis, the manner in which we interpret the signs and symbols within the sounds (Turino 2008). While these signs and symbols have been interpreted by scholars in search of the meanings within the sonorous properties of music and are often linked with style and genre (Meyer 1989; Monelle 2000; Hatten 2004), they may equally become associated with different situations, occasions, activities, locations, or identities, and thus contextualize the spaces in which they are heard. It is these signs and the atmospheres that they can help to cultivate that regulate and structure our everyday lives.

Since this chapter discusses the application of audiovisual media to influence behavior, I draw from theories around the encoding and decoding of media texts (Hall 1973) in order to analyze some of the symbols and cues that can be found in the music video. In one of these approaches, musicologist Nicholas Cook (2001) applies a form of reception theory to the discussion of audiovisual texts, in the form of television commercials, among other things. Drawing from Miller's (1987) work on material culture, Cook argues that what he calls attributes, which are the characteristics of an object or text and the potential meanings encoded within them, are interpreted by audience members in a process he refers to as actualization. This, he suggests, helps to account for the polysemic nature of audiovisual media. By actualizing a quantity of a text's indefinite number of attributes, Cook argues, each audience member creates an individualized account of what a particular text means to them and thus decodes the text in a manner particular to their own personal and sociocultural contexts.

The "ZAZI" music video presents four scenes in which women make healthy and positive life choices. These mini-narratives feed into a broader plot, in which Zonke leads an ever-growing crowd of women and girls toward a performance space that is shown at various points throughout the video. Wearing a flowing green dress, the singer walks up to a fence outside a pink house that is slightly out of focus in the background and ties a green ribbon around the fencepost. The instrumentation in the introduction is important. A clean electric guitar opens the track with a wah-wah-inflected riff before the introduction of the drum kit, synthesized bass, and Hammond organ.[1] The dramatic and shimmering organ glissando and subsequent improvisations mark the end of the instrumental introduction. The relatively slow tempo—roughly 90 bpm—and embellishing bass guitar grooves give the track a relaxed and funky quality.

For Meintjes (2003), the Hammond organ is "distinctly associated with the sound of soul" (136). South African soul has its roots in African American soul, which in turn grew out of gospel (Werner 2006). As is the case in South Africa, the songs and sounds of the African American civil rights movement were heavily influenced by the hymns and gospel songs of African American churches, from which many Black pastors preached their revolutionary rhetoric (Calhoun-Brown 2000). James Brown, the legendary Godfather of soul, is noted to have remarked that soul and the Black civil rights movement could not be separated from one another in the United States (Werner 2006). The development of soul music in the United States was very much intertwined with gospel songs and the rhetoric of praise and love that accompanied them. Indeed, in the early 1960s, some scholars suggested it was difficult to distinguish between the two genres (Maultsby 2005).

Presenting ZAZI through the genre of Afro-soul potentially constructs a connection between the messages and the associated meanings coded within that genre, something that Cook (1994) would refer to as the transferal of attributes from the music to the message. In this instance, for example, the meanings coded within the soul genre generally and the Hammond organ specifically, may include faith, community, resistance, struggle, and the divine, through African American gospel music and civil rights movements in the United States and South Africa. It is worth being very clear from the outset, however, that audiences are not passive entities and each interpretation of the music video will ultimately be based on cultural, social, and individual experiences and identities (Levine 2007). Given that the ZAZI campaign seeks to influence opinions and attitudes around women's empowerment and health, as was mentioned in previous chapters in the discussions of both the TAC movement and music in advertising, any association with human rights struggles is likely to help legitimize and protect ZAZI's messaging.

In the video's opening scene, Zonke walks along a path between fields of tall, dry, yellow grass that appears golden in the low evening sunlight. In the background, a dim mountain landscape contrasts against the paling sky. The viewer is then transported into an urban setting. Zonke moves toward a little girl in a dress and ties another green ribbon to the girl's bicycle before walking away, with the girl following. The organ and guitar interact with complementing blues-style flattened seventh mixolydian melodies over an upbeat I-VII-IV harmonic progression played by the bass and piano. The use of flattened seventh melodies is typical of blues, soul, and rhythm and blues, and further underscores the track's associations with the music of Black America in times of struggle for agency and dignity. The music video presents women and girls of all ages and many of South Africa's ethnicities.

> Hey girl, we know it's hard sometimes
> You feeling lost somehow, cannot see the signs
>
> (Zonke Dikana, "ZAZI," Joe Public, Johannesburg, 2013)

In the first scene, an older man sits alone in his car playing with a gold lighter as he watches a girl's netball game, ominously licking his lips as he does so. A small crowd has gathered to watch them play, but the man does not appear to be part of it, choosing instead to watch from a distance.

> It seems lonely, but you've got strength inside
> But you've got strength inside to leave it all behind 'Cause you know who you are
>
> (Zonke Dikana, "ZAZI," Joe Public, Johannesburg, 2013)

The lyrics "It seems lonely, but you've got strength inside" then emphasize inner strength, with the video alluding to physical prowess through the girl's netball match. An adolescent girl celebrates what appear to be points scored as the ball bounces off toward the lone man, who is now outside, leaning on his car. As the ball rolls to his feet, we see that he is very well dressed with many signs of wealth and status, including a gold watch, smart clothing and shoes, sunglasses, and a gold lighter.

> Don't know where to go, vision's getting blurry
> Don't see nobody to turn to
>
> (Zonke Dikana, "ZAZI," Joe Public, Johannesburg, 2013)

The man picks up the ball as the young girl jogs over to collect it, but the man does not offer it to her, and instead he looks her up and down in her athletic skirt and T-shirt. The young girl then grabs the ball from him, giving him a stern and disapproving look as she walks away, leaving the older man visibly shocked at her response. A teammate gives the girl a high-five and spins her around before removing a green ribbon from her hair and tying it to the original girl's wrist.

> Look inside you, you'll know what you're about
> Just let it show, ZAZI who you are.
>
> (Zonke Dikana, "ZAZI," Joe Public, Johannesburg, 2013)

The chorus retains the harmonic structure of the verses while the piano plays the progression in a staccato manner. The melody places great emphasis on the opening phrase, which is encompassed entirely by the lyrics "ZAZI" illustrating the importance of the Nguni phrase, meaning "know yourself." The track's dynamics fade slightly during the chorus, and the timbre of Zonke's vocals becomes soft and breathy, as if attempting to soothe someone.

> ZAZI, it's time to know yourself
> You know you got the strength, ZAZI who you are.
>
> (Zonke Dikana, "ZAZI," Joe Public, Johannesburg, 2013)

Indeed, much of the song could be considered to be directed at a specific person. The dynamic change does not seem anti-climactic due to the inclusion of punchy piano chords and clean mixolydian guitar fills.

> ZAZI, it's time to love yourself
> You know you got the strength, ZAZI who you are.
>
> (Zonke Dikana, "ZAZI," Joe Public, Johannesburg, 2013)

The netball team joins Zonke as she continues to walk and ties another green ribbon around a post. Throughout the video, increasing numbers of women follow Zonke, in her flowing robe-like dress, toward the final performance space. As the netball team follows Zonke, they walk several meters behind her through the golden glowing fields. The video cuts to evening scenes of Zonke performing a small rooftop concert to young women.

> So keep it going, just keep it moving on
> 'Cause life is better when you know who you are.
>
> (Zonke Dikana, "ZAZI," Joe Public, Johannesburg, 2013)

In the second scene, a young woman, presumably a student, sits alone at a dining room table covered with books as she reads and makes notes on a particular text. She looks at her phone before her attention is drawn to a group of young women in a convertible Mini Cooper waiting outside.

> Your choices matter, whether big or small
> No it don't take that long to look inside you
>
> (Zonke Dikana, "ZAZI," Joe Public, Johannesburg, 2013)

As the student appears at her door, the group of women begin ushering her to join them. She smiles but shakes her head, and the others shrug before moving along. As the young student returns to her books, she opens one to find a green ribbon waiting for her. She ties it to her pen as a man enters the scene to bring her a cup of tea.

> Let's keep this going
> You matter, let nobody say you don't

(Zonke Dikana, "ZAZI," Joe Public, Johannesburg, 2013)

The track then breaks into a refrain in which backing vocals sing a cyclical riff as Zonke repeats important lyrical motifs such as "you got the strength in you" while decorating the interlude with vocal embellishments.

> Look inside you and you'll know
> You got the strength in you (got the strength in you)

(Zonke Dikana, "ZAZI," Joe Public, Johannesburg, 2013)

In the third scene, a woman who appears to be in her twenties sits in a family planning clinic while a nurse displays a packet of contraceptive pills. The nurse further discusses female condoms as she places one into a bag and hands it to the young woman. A conservatively dressed older woman appears from the background of the scene and looks disapprovingly at the exchange between the young woman and the nurse, as more (now male) condoms are placed into the bag. As she turns to leave the clinic, she is stopped by the older woman, who smiles, removes her green scarf, and places it around the young woman's neck. The crowd continues to follow Zonke as she walks into a town center and ties a ribbon around a traffic light pole.

The final scene depicts a couple arguing in a car while rain lashes against the windows. The man shouts while gesticulating and points aggressively toward what appears to be his partner. The woman's gaze begins to glaze over as she tunes out the barrage of aggression. She seems to refocus her attention away from her partner and toward herself. As the walking crowd of women following Zonke appear in the scene, the woman abruptly gets out of the car, much to her partner's surprise. She takes off a green ribbon she had been wearing as a belt, wraps it around a nearby lamppost, and raises her arms into the rain before joining the rest of the women and girls walking with Zonke.

King Nova, a South African poet, recites her poetry over the chorus, which repeats at a reduced volume in the background, reminding those listening to know and love themselves.

Know yourself as the true compass
Where blessed beginnings are first born

(King Nova in Zonke Dikana, "ZAZI," Joe Public, Johannesburg, 2013)

In the scenes prior to reciting her poem, Nova is seen presenting her clenched fists to the camera, and on her fingers, she is wearing rings in the shape of birds. The clenched fist has become synonymous around the world with the struggle for human and civil rights, and in South Africa, it is an important signifier of the liberation struggle (Badat 1999). Indeed, the first line of Nova's poem alludes to signifying strength: "You symbolize the strength of every woman who has ever had to walk this road." Encoded within these scenes is the ongoing struggle for women's rights through the application of a well-known struggle symbol, over a musical chorus that encourages women to know and love themselves.

The women and girls that have been following Zonke now appear in the rooftop concert that the singer has been performing throughout each scene. The video pans away and fades out as all the women and girls clap together and sing the song's chorus a cappella. The allusion to the choir trope, though slightly subtler than other examples that can be found in humanitarian anthems, intimates that ZAZI may potentially not be so far removed from the Band Aid formula of celebrity campaigning discussed in Chapter 5. Throughout the video, Zonke leads the women and girls from each scene toward the rooftop performance space. In the finale, we see that there is no distinction between the musicians and the audience, insofar as there are women and girls both on stage with Zonke and in the audience area. The sense of unity encoded within the finale is further intensified during the final repetition of the main line of the chorus, as all instrumentation and amplification is cut and the whole crowd sings in harmony.

Each of the scenes was designed to inspire women to make similar choices when presented with such decisions. Role modeling indeed plays an important part in many edutainment campaigns (Somers 2008; Tufte 2008), but what "ZAZI" ultimately seeks to capitalize on is the strong mobilizing effect music and imagery can engender through various cues and references to powerful emotional stimuli such as the liberation struggle, unity, and spiritual sentiments. The scenes that play out within the music video contribute to a wider narrative of women's agency in the choices that they make. During our interview, one of the creative directors of the "ZAZI" music video noted the importance of the story within "ZAZI."

> It was very very specific that we wanted to target the heartstrings and we needed the kind of people and the kind of genre and music that could help us to tell a story, but to tell a beautiful story, an uplifting story. But not to do something that was just there for the sake of being. It had to have meaning. That is how we ended up where we did from an artist point of view as well as a genre point of view. We wanted to situate the campaign in a familiar but also contemporary style, one that speaks to what it means to be a South African. (Interview with creative team members behind the "ZAZI" music video, March 2014)

The familiarity that was noted is likely a reference to the long history of South Africa's oral traditions. Narratives have been woven by traditional Xhosa and Zulu storytellers for generations. These *ingoma* (songs) and *iintsomi* (folktales) have been used to teach children about their culture, maintain social harmony, resolve conflicts, and instill moral education (McNeill 2011; Neethling 1990). These practices, however, are not separate. In the world of *iintsomi*, narratives are developed through drama, dance, mime, songs, and chants, before the storyteller recounts their tale (Morris 1989). Fittingly, the "ZAZI" music video appears to pay homage to these traditional roots. *Iintsomi* have typically been thematically concerned with conflict—often in the form of jealousy, violence, or social unrest within families or communities—and resolution. The stories highlight individual or social shortcomings and provide solutions to problems while furnishing them with the moral authority of wisdom and experience.

Music, Lyrics, and Image: Marketing Education as Entertainment

What is immediately noticeable about the "ZAZI" song is that it makes no direct reference to any of the campaign goals, opting instead to present positive messages about knowing and loving oneself. This is an unusual departure from the standard model of music-driven campaigning, which tends to be quite transparent with the subject matter. During our interview, Bronwyn touched upon some of the reasoning behind that creative decision.

> What is at the heart of the challenges that young women face, given that we live in a fairly patriarchal society? A lot of areas in South Africa are very traditional still. We know that some women will do well, they'll succeed, they'll break out of that cycle. But what is that one thing that breaks you out or keeps you in the

> cycle? A lot of women would say to us: it's about self-esteem. (Interview with Bronwyn Pierce, February 2014)

These messages of self-esteem are found throughout the lyrics, with specific examples transmitted visually through four separate scenes in which women and girls make positive life choices when faced with common issues for many South Africans such as domestic violence, education, transactional relationships or "sugar daddies," and sexual health. By removing direct references from the lyrics, the "ZAZI" song does not have to contend with numerous complex and nuanced issues in its lyrics. Celebrities are often accused of oversimplifying or misrepresenting humanitarian or public health issues (Huliaras and Tzifakis 2012), with some analysts and scholars describing the depth of understanding presented by even the most renowned of celebrity activists as "breathtakingly one-dimensional" (Dieter and Kumar 2008, 259). Perhaps one of the biggest challenges facing health and humanitarian campaign songs is the limited ways in which people can meaningfully connect with such lyrics. The ZAZI campaign's approach avoids presenting specific one-dimensional messages.

By drawing from both the audio and visual resources available within the video format, "ZAZI" is able to present itself as something outside of the standard mold of music video campaigning. Since the scenes are brief and without dialogue, one might well argue that they themselves simplify complex issues. However, as musicologist Carol Vernallis (2004) explains, "[i]f the intent of a music video lies in drawing attention to the music—whether to provide commentary upon it or simply to sell it—it makes sense that the image ought not to carry a story or plot in the way that a film might" (3–4). Indeed, the scenes are designed to do exactly that, to draw attention to and complement the coded messages of strength and self-worth presented in the music. She notes that each element of the multimedia experience (music, lyrics, and image) "possess their own language with regard to time, space, narrativity, activity, and affect" (2004, 13).

The use of short but poignant visual segments in "ZAZI," depicting issues that are likely to have been experienced by large numbers of young women and girls, would theoretically encourage them to engage more readily with the message. Pink (2006) notes a similar theme in Susan Levine's work on documentary film in HIV/AIDS awareness. She argues that Levine's work "demonstrated how people's base-line knowledge [. . .] increased after viewing locally produced films that they could engage with at a level of narrative and individual experience"

(91). According to Pink, then, such engagement with individual experience may facilitate engagement with the audiovisual material.

Despite the importance of visual narratives, however, it was the music, rather than the visuals, that the ZAZI campaign hoped would be the catalyst for social change and awareness of women's sexual health concerns. This can be inferred from the way in which one of the creative team describes how they came to the idea of using music as their chosen catalyst for change:

> When we decided to go with music we thought: listen, girls really really respond well to music and it's also a matter of how do you take a somewhat taboo subject matter and actually make it palatable, and dare we say funky? So it was around that time that we decided "okay guys, let's create an anthem, let's create a song, something that will be able to get to the heart of the issues that women across South Africa face." (Interview with creative team members behind the "ZAZI" music video, March 2014)

It is apparent that the "ZAZI" creators and organizers understood that music could be used as a tool to communicate about subjects that may be socially unpalatable. By using a song, or an anthem as it was described, the creative team hoped to not only create a discussion about women's rights in South Africa but also attempt to challenge the social stigma around gender norms and socially taboo subjects such as gender-based violence. It became clearer, as we continued to discuss the use of music as a campaigning tool, that organizers are often aware that music or songs may be a useful way of engaging people meaningfully with a subject, but perhaps less aware of the mechanics of such processes. As a ubiquitous mass-media commodity and social activity, music presents an effective vehicle for disseminating messages to large numbers of people (Singhal and Rogers 2012), but campaign organizers largely do not engage in discussions of how music has been shown to be effective at mobilizing mass action generally, and in South Africa particularly. Put simply, they are aware of the "what" of music in campaigning, but not necessarily the "how."

A further important point to consider is how the lyrics of "ZAZI" influence the reception of the song. Describing edutainment more generally, Greenberg et al. (2004) note that ensuring the two components of the portmanteau (education and entertainment) are virtually indistinguishable from one another is paramount to its success. During my interview with Bronwyn, we touched upon the importance of creating entertaining content as a matter of priority.

> Often we [Johns Hopkins] choose something like a drama series, or commercials, or whatever, but in this instance we chose music specifically because we believe that when you put messaging out there, it needs to be entertaining. If it's not entertaining, you've already lost the battle. So, for us it is about entertainment and how do we use that element of entertainment to basically get identification with the campaign. (Interview with Bronwyn Pierce, February 2014)

By removing direct references to the campaign goals from the lyrics, the "ZAZI" track becomes less distinguishable as a campaign song and is therefore not faced with the same challenges of creating entertaining and marketable content from public health messages as other music-driven initiatives. ZAZI is able to market itself as a more approachable form of campaigning, situated toward the consumer-friendly "entertainment" end of the edutainment spectrum. The catchy and upbeat song, sung by a popular up-and-coming South African pop singer, gains much of the marketability of a regular pop song while simultaneously retaining the meanings and connotations of the four scenes illustrating women making healthy, self-respecting, and considered lifestyle choices.

HIV/AIDS "Clutter" in the South African Media Landscape

The use of mass media within health and humanitarian campaigning is well-documented (Ray and Donohew 1990; Backer, Rogers, and Sopory 1992; Donovan and Henley 2010; Sidahmed, Soderlund, and Briggs 2010). Across the African continent, various HIV-related initiatives have utilized television, radio, music, documentary film, or social media in an attempt to raise awareness and prevent further infections (Levine 2007; van Buren 2011; Breitinger 2011). In South Africa, however, media platforms have been particularly overburdened with, at times conflicting, AIDS-related messages and calls to action from various sources. This presents an additional barrier to effective HIV/AIDS awareness raising. Messaging from multiple sources, each with their own ideas on how best to tackle AIDS-related issues, has the potential to deeply confuse the narratives around the disease. Further, given the sheer extent of media coverage, and the number of initiatives that have dealt with AIDS in South Africa, it is unsurprising that indifference to the epidemic presents a significant hurdle for health communicators. During our interview, Bronwyn highlighted this as a concern for the ZAZI campaign.

> Often, I think, when you do a campaign like this, especially a health campaign, it's often staged and boring. People don't really connect with some of the messaging and some of the communication we do around health, especially HIV and AIDS. We've learned over time that when a campaign is identified as an HIV campaign, immediately people are really sort of put off by it. I think there's a lot of, sort of, fatigue around HIV and AIDS messaging because we've been doing it for so long in South Africa. There's definitely a little bit of fatigue so, you know, developing something that young women can identify with and own, basically, is really important. (Interview with Bronwyn Pierce, February 2014)

While the subject of the Mbeki government's unenthusiastic responses to the emerging AIDS crisis has been covered earlier in this book, it is worth restating the profound influence of such inaction and state-sponsored AIDS dissidence on the collective South African consciousness. Issues relating to apathy, denial, misconception, and stigma that continued long after the end of his administration can largely be attributed to the denialism perpetuated under his leadership (Visser and Sipsma 2013).

Given the onslaught of misinformation and AIDS anti-science that characterized this period of the South African AIDS crisis, it is unsurprising that there has been a high volume of educational media addressing the issue, the vast majority of which is in the form of mass-media campaigning. Indeed, such is the extent of South Africa's HIV/AIDS media clutter that scholarship is emerging to suggest, as Bronwyn noted, that people are beginning to tune out the messages relating to HIV/AIDS (Walker 2022b). While discussing this with Bronwyn, not only was she acutely aware of the wealth of AIDS-related media available in the country but also further attempted to distance "ZAZI" from other campaign music videos.

> I think for us, the music isn't the campaign. The music was basically a vehicle. Our challenge in South Africa, even though we are an African country, is that we have a lot of media clutter, it's difficult to break through, that's always our challenge. We have a lot of work going on in South Africa around HIV and AIDS; there are a lot of people doing a lot of different things. So, music was just a way for us to, for one, position the campaign, to get that appeal and pull people into the campaign. So, it isn't the campaign and there are many other formats in which we deliver the campaign, with music being one of those. In terms of launching the campaign and putting it out into the public domain, music was the vehicle we chose to do that. (Interview with Bronwyn Pierce, February 2014)

For Bronwyn, then, the "ZAZI" music video was used as a way to draw as many people as possible into the campaign and attempt to invigorate a somewhat stale discussion.

Transient Pseudo-Effervescence in Audiovisual Interventions

So far in this chapter, I have discussed the "ZAZI" music video in abstract terms and often in relation to its production. In order to better understand the effect that music videos may have on those who experience them, I set up a small screening of the "ZAZI" music video for young South Africans, a key demographic that the campaign seeks to influence. I did so by reaching out to high schools and further education colleges that provide educational opportunities to some of Cape Town's most underprivileged areas. One of those schools was happy to facilitate this experiment as part of the students' ongoing HIV/AIDS education in their Life Orientation classes. The approach was very simple: the students would fill out a brief questionnaire that explored their opinions relating to the video and its messages as they were viewing it. Shortly after the screenings, the students would be divided into groups to discuss their opinions in more detail in focus groups, if they wished to do so.

It is mid-morning when I arrive at the school, and the student participants are already filing into the main assembly hall. A school technician has set up the audiovisual equipment needed to screen the music video. After chatting briefly with the Life Orientation teacher about the schedule and format of events, I began to collect the parental consent forms that I had distributed a week prior. Upon counting the forms, it becomes clear that a small handful of students cannot participate, as they have forgotten to return their forms. When the final head count is done, there are an even 200 participants waiting to listen. After briefing them on the format of the study, I am assisted once again by their teacher to distribute the questionnaires.

The lights go down, and the opening guitar riff flows from the speakers as the image of Zonke Dikana in her striking green dress fades into view on the screen. Just as I had done so many times during the *Lucky, the Hero!* shows, I find a place toward the back of the hall to observe the screening, expecting to simply watch the music video with the participants. The students watch and listen with all eyes facing forward. Some are scribbling answers on their questionnaire papers, while others stare motionlessly at the screen. The first chorus comes and goes. Throughout the second verse, one of two people appear to have become distracted and begin chatting, while others still are attempting to hide their use of their phones from the teacher. But as the main hook repeats again for the second chorus, something starts to happen. As I look over the congregation of light blue-gray school uniforms, I notice that people have started to tap their feet and move their bodies in subtle ways to the beat and bass that is flowing through the formidable assembly hall speakers.

My eye is drawn to a small group of girls sitting at the front who have begun to sway to the music together in their seats. Others are now also showing the outward affective signs of musicking with small rhythmic gestures. Three more girls at the front have joined the group of swaying students, with some now moving their hips in their seats. They glance at one another and laugh. As the final chorus pours from the speakers, a low-level affective electricity appears to be spreading through the collection of participants. Some boys nod their heads or drum their fingers on their laps, while the number of learners moving their bodies subtly to the music has ballooned to encompass almost the first two rows of seats. The final a cappella lyrics of "ZAZI" resound through the hall as the track comes to a close and the motion dissipates.

Shortly after the song has ended and the lights have come back on, the students are divided into groups to discuss their perspectives about the music video. The responses were mixed. When asked about their opinions regarding the perceived influence of "ZAZI" on their future behavior, many of the students indicated that the song would have little to no effect on their daily lives.

> I don't think a video like that is going to change much. We know that there's a problem but people will see the video but then get on with their lives. (Female learner, aged 15–19, High School group interview 2015)

This sentiment was echoed by a number of other respondents across a spectrum of demographics such as gender, race, and age.

> What was the purpose? Are we supposed to be like the people in the video now? I don't know about anyone else but I don't feel like watching this video made any difference to how people will behave. (Male learner, aged 15–19, High School group interview 2015)

While responses like this seemed to indicate that the "ZAZI" song failed to influence those who listened to it, it was only when I began to work my way through the quantitative data gathered from the questionnaires that I noticed something that struck me as unusual. The results of the survey study seemed to show that the "ZAZI" music video was indeed effective, with 78 percent of respondents (156 students) indicating that they felt motivated toward improving women's rights in South Africa. Indeed, much of the survey data was encouraging for "ZAZI" with 69 percent of respondents (138 students) further noting a feeling of empowerment during the video.

These undeniably positive statistics contrast uncomfortably with the overwhelming consensus of the participants when the issue was discussed in the focus groups. How does one account for such radical departures from survey data collected from the same individuals only minutes earlier? It is important to remember that the participants were asked to fill in their questionnaires while they were listening to the "ZAZI" song and thus under the influence of its connective and affective properties. It seems that the students were engaged and motivated while watching the video and listening to the music, but that these feelings quickly faded once they had finished watching and listening to it. While the effect was limited, the affective displays among the participants are indicative of a transformation of the space from a regular assembly hall to one beginning to develop the kind of affectively charged atmosphere associated with musical effervescence.

The learners were experiencing heightened affective states, similar to those of participants of a *Lucky, the Hero!* show or a TAC march, albeit in a significantly less intense fashion. Durkheim's ([1912] 2008) understanding of religious fervor is built upon creating interpersonal connections between individuals. These connections then act as catalysts for the chain reaction between participants that culminates in effervescence. Music videos such as "ZAZI," however, present their information in a far more isolated manner, through pre-recorded performances to individuals or small groups of people within contexts that are often not conducive to effervescence such as television broadcasts, social media videos, or cell phone movie files. The heightened affective states discussed previously in this book are typically prolonged and sustained (as is the case with most emotional and affective phenomena) through contact with others, or in other words, through participation. The "ZAZI" music video, however, cultivated a counterfeit of musical effervescence, simulating some of its effects, but failing to ignite the same kinds of energy or electricity noted in previous chapters. This, I argue, is the same kind of phenomenon that motivated so many to donate to charitable causes as a result of Band Aid, USA for Africa, Artists Against Apartheid, and other celebrity supergroups: the Band Aid method of campaigning.

So, how does "ZAZI" engender a quasi-effervescent experience without achieving musical effervescence? The answer can be found in the students' responses. When asked about their dancing, the participants at the front of the hall noted that they felt the beat from the songs and decided to move to it.

> I don't normally listen to that kind of music but, after a while, I just started to feel into the beat. I saw some of my friends were also doing it, so I just went with it. I didn't feel like I was in class anymore, we don't really do this sort of thing much. It felt good. (Female learner, aged 15–19, High School group interview 2015)

The responses suggest that the students were affected by the music video. Their perception of the space was altered by the atmosphere cultivated by recorded music. Atmospheres are nebulous and affective environments. They involve feelings and emotions that transcend individual cognition or embodiment and instead refer to such feelings as they coalesce within a space (Riedel 2020). The most immediate aspects are felt through multi-sensorial stimulation and are interpreted in largely unconscious and pre-discursive ways. Comprehension of these atmospheres is an altogether slower process than the initial affective response as it leverages prior associations and learned behaviors to provide social and emotional context to the experience (McGraw 2016).

For many scholars of music and performance, there is no such thing as passive listening, since the act of listening requires a great deal from the human body and mind (Cavicchi 2002; Schechner 2004). Indeed, interpretation of affective cues employs frames of reference that are deeply embedded in our social and cultural worldviews and, as such, seem innate to the surroundings. Music often plays a particularly prominent role in creating and maintaining these atmospheric conditions, filling spaces with indefinite interpretational possibilities. While we may not always be aware of the causes, wherever music resonates, we are subject to encountering feelings in whatever ways our experiential memory may render it meaningful.

The experience of transient pseudo-effervescence can be a very powerful one, as exemplified by the money raised by similar pseudo-effervescent campaigns such as Band Aid and USA for Africa, and thus the respondents—who were watching the "ZAZI" video as they completed the survey—would have answered according to their feelings and emotions at that moment. What is striking is the speed at which those feelings of motivation elicited by "ZAZI" change. The effect begins to diminish almost immediately after the song or music video has ended. One student who insightfully inquired, "What was the purpose?" unearthed the core of the problem. The roughly three-minute and forty-five-second song is simply not long enough or impactful enough for individuals to make a meaningful connection with the purpose—a fundamental component of musical effervescence. While the video does present a series of short scenes that provide the opportunity for narrative interpretation, they are missing the kind of character investment and development found in the *Lucky, the Hero!* shows. Without a robust connection to a purpose, the process of cultivating musical effervescence fails.

Despite this, it would be wrong to suggest that a form of effervescence does not apply. Transient pseudo-effervescence extends Durkheim's theory of collective effervescence to encompass the kinds of quasi-effervescent expressions and experiences elicited by the "ZAZI" music video. It can be thought of as a momentarily euphoric or affective experience elicited through mass-media audiovisual stimuli that is directed toward a particular moral purpose. As campaign music videos are often accompanied by a call to action of some description, pseudo-effervescence becomes an important phenomenon in mobilizing such action. The term is used in this chapter more specifically to describe the phenomenon of fleeting mobilization toward specific campaign objectives while exposed to related motivational media. In some forms, it can be a powerful motivator, such as within the campaigns associated with the supergroups noted earlier, but the experience fades from the forefront of the mind almost as soon as the motivational media has ceased. Our emotional connections with recorded music are more often than not short-lived and unmemorable (Sloboda 2010). At times, music may elicit negative responses such as irritation, but often this too is fleeting and passes as quickly as the music does. The transience of the recorded musical experience by and large seems to lead to equally transient emotional states.

Campaign anthems and music videos represent the final applications of songs for HIV/AIDS-related positive health and social outcomes discussed in this book. The "ZAZI" music video, coupled with the historical successes—at least in monetary terms—of celebrity advocacy discussed in Chapter 5, shows that it is possible to engage participants in a limited capacity through an audiovisual mass-media format. However, transient pseudo-effervescence, missing a strong connection with a purpose, as well as interactive and participatory elements, fails to achieve the kinds of manic creativity associated with musical effervescence. As a result, effervescence-like qualities of music videos are lost the moment the audiovisual experience ends, surviving only within the fleeting affective qualities of music in the moment.

Note

1 "Wah-wah" is an onomatopoeic term used to describe the use of spectral glides to modify the vowel quality of a pitch. The resultant sound imitates the sound of a person saying the vowels "wah wah" (/ˈwɑː.wɑː/) and is commonly associated with the trombone and electric guitar.

10

Consequent

The Songs of the South African AIDS Crisis

Standing at the back of an expansive community hall, I do my best to prepare my recording equipment with icy and numb fingers. It is mid-winter and I am in the small Free State town of Hlohlolwane setting up my camera to document a *Lucky, the Hero!* performance for members of the Community Work Programme (CWP).[1] The old and slightly dilapidated town hall still has a certain majesty to it, despite falling into disrepair. Whatever its original purpose, it still retains a sense of grandeur. The place is frigid. My breath condenses the moment it leaves my body and rises in slow misty columns. Strip blinds billow in the draft of broken windows and peeled paint dusts the scratched and broken hardwood floor. Upon arrival about half an hour earlier, I took a few moments to explore the interior, partly to look for a better angle to shoot from and partly to explore this regal old building. I eventually found myself up in the stalls. Below me, men in hats and gloves are now setting out rusty metal chairs missing much of their foam cushioning, as bars of brilliant morning sunlight strike through the hall from high narrow windows, temporarily illuminating streams of tranquil dust suspended in the still air.

My mind wanders in the cold, perhaps in an attempt to keep itself warm with a mental brisk walk. I think back to one of the many discussions I had with Professor Jimmie Earl Perry. He would often ponder out loud some of the deeper questions that related to his work as a humanitarian, ardent HIV/AIDS advocate, and goodwill ambassador. During one of our chats, he spoke at length about his views on the ways in which music can be rendered meaningful, and how this might be applied to the health crisis.

> It doesn't matter if you're in Mpumalanga in a village or here in the urbanized Cape Town, everyone will know certain songs and they'll react to it. If a lyric

> has a meaning that affects you in any kind of way then it can be considered impactive. (Personal conversation with Prof Jimmie Earl Perry, 2014)

He leans back in his chair as a slight intensity flashes across his eyes. Raising his hands before him in expressive gesticulation, his many metal bangles and bracelets provide a tinkling and jingling accompaniment to his oration.

> The power and meanings in songs are found right the way through them. When your feet are moving, and your hands are clapping, or you're doing a chicken neck dance, as well as processing whatever the lyrics are, they're all going to work simultaneously to give an even stronger impact on what it means to you, and how you'll respond to it. (Personal conversation with Prof Jimmie Earl Perry, 2014)

After a moment of silence, a short burst of laughter resonates from the professor, noticing his own animated clapping and jingling.

> Let me put it like this, everyone is going to have a different opinion on what makes them tick when they hear a certain beat, lyric, or voice, everyone will react slightly differently. But I would wager this, they will react and that reaction will be contagious. (Personal conversation with Prof Jimmie Earl Perry, 2014)

The temperate Stellenbosch afternoon snaps back to Hlohlolwane's winter as shrill yelling from a somehow aggrieved technician brings me back into the cold reality of the community hall. Warm breath momentarily brings some feeling back into my clasped hands as I tighten a clasp on my camera stand. As I watch from my perch in the stalls, workers in orange uniforms trickle in, and before long the hall echoes with scraping chairs, movement, and Sotho chattering. The lights go up, and the chattering fades as the theater company open their first performance of the day.

The CWP participants are enthralled throughout the participatory performance. They roar with laughter as Two-Time Tokie peacocks his way into the audience and they shout impromptu responses to the quasi-rhetorical questions posed by the main character, Lucky, as he throws his exaggerated oration playfully toward the crowd. It is a narrative of HIV/AIDS awareness and acceptance that, after over a year of tagging along to various performances across the country, I am now well acquainted with. After nearly an hour, momentum starts to build toward the finale, and I see subtle gestures of anticipation from the audience: glances around the room, shifting in seats, and sporadic outbursts of clapping or shouting.

The soft and breathy sound of the actors' voices reverberates up toward the rafters as they set up for the grand finale, their voices echoing slightly on the reflective whitewashed walls of the once grand hall. The final anticipatory pitch is held by the collection of voices for a moment, agonizingly long for those expecting the immediate satisfaction of musical resolution, until a thumping dance beat explodes from the sound system, igniting the potential energy of the room. The singers step from side to side, clapping to the beat while singing with full accompaniment provided by the booming PA system. By the time the musical finale is in full swing, most of the participants are already on their feet, inhibitions thrown to the wayside, moving their bodies to the high-tempo pulse, as a syncopated digital brass section punctuates the melody of a reimagined version of "I Will Survive." Some dance alone, while others feverishly encourage others to join them. I watch as a small number of women at the front begin to dance their way closer to the actors. Ricardo, who plays the character Lucky, moves forward to meet them, throwing his hands in the air beside them while continuing an impressively melismatic phrase over the accompanying harmonies.

This phenomenon—one that I have witnessed dozens of times—usually begins with a small cell of dancers at the front of the audience and spreads throughout the participants until they are all on their feet, caught in the euphoria of music, dance, and shared emotional energy. But just as the final participants at the back of the hall have lost their inhibitions, the song is over. As the last notes of the finale fade from the speakers, the coordinator of the CWP, an easy-going Sotho man in a casual jacket, jeans, and shoulder-length dreadlocks, is handed a microphone and immediately shouts "do you want to hear that again!?" Everyone is surprised since the previously agreed-upon plan was for him to ask for volunteers to come up and talk about the show or their experiences of HIV/AIDS. The audience unanimously cheers in agreement for an encore of the final song. The theater group, who are not immune to their own methods of creating affectively charged environments of musical effervescence, are more than happy to oblige. As the beat of "I Will Survive" once again pumps through the PA system, everyone in the hall springs back to their feet, instantly reviving the electric energy of a few moments earlier.

The song comes to its climactic end to rapturous applause. Many women continue dancing regardless, and as the theater group are leaving the performance area, one of the actors suddenly jumps upon a fellow peer educator and throws her arms around her in glee before leaving the stage. As I pan my camera back and forth, taking in the spectacle as best I can, the above words from a casual conversation with Professor Perry repeat in my mind. People seem to lose themselves within the moment, and in that moment, inhibitions are lost, new relationships are cultivated between strangers, and socially constructed paradigms of behavior break down. The reactions are spontaneous, invigorating, impactful, contagious, and very real.

Contributions and Limitations

In some ways, I have strayed from the conventional norms and protocols of ethnomusicological and anthropological scholarship around AIDS in Africa. While authors in these fields typically focus attention on detailed and in-depth accounts of communities, groups, or organizations (see McNeill 2011; Barz 2006, Okigbo 2016; Black 2019), I have sought in this book to examine a seemingly disparate selection of songs and singers from across the country that demonstrate the diversity of music-related HIV/AIDS interventions, broadly conceived. However, questions of how and why songs became such a ubiquitous and formidable force within the South African AIDS epidemic are connected to much broader themes related to music in human life.

As I noted in Chapter 3, a growing body of evidence indicates that music—and particularly singing—is woven into what it means to be human. This book has drawn from a wealth of interdisciplinary theoretical tools to develop an approach that grounds interpersonal musical experiences—and the heightened affective states that often accompany them—in our shared human journey of development as a species. By doing so, I frame such encounters as fundamental expressions of shared humanity, whose bonds may cultivate synchronicities of movement, perception, experience, and perspective. In short, this book connects the variety of interventions discussed within these pages through a phenomenological approach to musical experiences—particularly collective singing—that I have called musical effervescence. Musical effervescence helps to explain how songs are able to be so many different things to different people at the same time, yet foreground a shared humanity that is often able to transcend our many divisions.

Durkheim's collective effervescence describes the social forces that determine heightened states of being generated by collecting in large numbers. While his theory of crowd behavior continues to be relevant today, Durkheim's model only gestures toward what my observations suggest is a crucial component of creating and maintaining this phenomenon. While music is not the only medium through which to cultivate effervescence, it is highly effective and expedites the process of synchronizing individuals into a collective through rhythm, pulse, and affective sonorous components. As demonstrated throughout this book, whether in a *Lucky, the Hero!* performance among Free State high school students, HIV-positive choirs, or national activist organizations, the musical elements observed by Durkheim ([1912] 2008) are not simply relegated to "order permitting cooperation" (216). The emotional and kinetic energy released through musical effervescence is harnessed by these groups for varying purposes, each of which has been shown to have improved health and social outcomes.

The primary questions to understanding musical effervescence are "who is singing and for what purpose?," "what is the music doing?," and "what is the music not doing?" The flow chart provided in Chapter 3 helps to summarize what the music is doing. It is channeling musicking with a purpose through heightened affected states of intersubjectivity and synchronicity of bodies and minds into forms of manic creativity, within which participants may conceptualize new social relationships and realities related to the purpose. But it is equally important to understand what the music is not doing. In the examples of the 46664 AIDS benefit concerts discussed in Chapter 5 and the "ZAZI" music video discussed in Chapter 9, signifiers of musical effervescence seem to be present among the participating groups (whether participants who are watching the music video or audiences within the stadiums). One might reasonably suggest that a stadium concert is a prime location for high-energy musical experiences that resemble musical effervescence. But these examples are missing key components that are necessary for musical effervescence as a transformative musical experience.

The 46664 benefit concerts were missing purpose—an immediacy to the cause—and participation—an immediacy to the performance, insofar as the presentational nature of the concerts limited how audiences became involved with and shaped the performance. The "ZAZI" music video suffered similar deficiencies. As an audiovisual intervention, embodiment, synchronicity, participation, and proximity are largely absent. Moreover, the purpose behind the intervention is one step further removed from the prospective participants than it would have been in a live performance—which as we have seen in the 46664 concerts, is itself no guarantee of musical effervescence. Thus, proximity to other individuals is dependent on the nature of the viewing experience, and proximity to the performative elements of the musicking experience is mediated by way of audiovisual recording and therefore distant.

In instances such as those with the 46664 concerts and the "ZAZI" music video, in which effervescence appears to be present but lacks the kind of manic creativity that is the hallmark of musical effervescence, a form of transient pseudo-effervescence emerges. This is defined as a brief heightened affective state facilitated through music that dissipates immediately when the music ends and does not facilitate forms of manic creativity through which ideal forms of social relationships may emerge. It is simply affective and emotional arousal via music in the moment. However, this is not to say that these transient experiences cannot influence behavior in those moments. The money raised by Live Aid and Band Aid illustrates the degree to which people under the influence of transient pseudo-effervescence can be compelled to take certain actions—in this case, to make donations.

This does, however, raise questions regarding the *Lucky, the Hero!* shows, which also have a significant presentational element to the performance but are often able to cultivate musical effervescence among the participants of the intervention. In this case, it helps to acknowledge that the *Lucky, the Hero!* performances are not exclusively musical events. While sonic embodiment is structured through strategically placed live amplified pop music and participatory interludes, the Educational Theatre Company is also able to quickly build connections between the characters and their needs—or purpose—and the audience by employing musical theater approaches such as role modeling and narrative to their intervention. By encouraging the audience to invest in the characters' development and the calculated application of audience interactions, the actors are often able to cultivate a vicarious sense of purpose that becomes realized through engendering an immediacy between the subject matter and the audience that culminates in the highly participatory musical finale of the show.

Finally, the TAC activists drew extensively from the mobilizing and energizing properties of musical effervescence in part due to the urgency of their situation. Their lives and/or the lives of their friends and loved ones depended on making ARV therapies available to everyone who needed them through the South African public health service. This urgency of purpose and the dangers associated with living openly with HIV at a time when activists were at significant risk of physical violence as a result of their HIV status provided the fuel for a frenetic energy that was channeled into their collective musicking, culminating in powerful displays of musical effervescence and manic creativity.

Given the breadth of examples provided in this book, it is clear that musical effervescence cannot be characterized by a single event or experience. There is certainly more than one way to achieve this state. One might expect to see and hear effervescent displays in all manner of musicking with purpose, including protests, religious events, or performative rituals, to name a few. Shared experiences and manifestations emerge as a consequence of being together in music. By exploring the roots of musical effervescence deep within humanity's own evolutionary story, this book has positioned the songs of the South African AIDS crisis not only as a profoundly human response to the greatest public health catastrophe in South Africa's history, but also as fundamental tools in the disparate struggles against HIV (for health, life, awareness, social acceptance, etc.) and musical effervescence as a powerful force for health and healing.

In this book, I have attempted to balance representations regarding the importance of the cultural influence of music with a clearly framed theoretical model of musically situated intersubjectivity that is applicable across various contexts. It is evident that the importance of songs and other performing arts within South African cultures and identity bears influence on the phenomenon of musical effervescence. As Professor Perry noted in the vignette that introduces this chapter, the "power and meanings in songs are found right the way through them." This power and meaning are often situated within a cultural framework that renders meaningful the sonorous qualities of music. Indeed, those songs that energized participants to embodied forms of affective expression would likely have failed to do so if there were no culturally understood systems, however nebulous and dynamic, of musical meanings.

In South Africa in particular, the application of music and songs as a cultural tool for important aspects of everyday life such as social cohesion, education, initiation, or celebration, existed long before colonial settlers introduced western tertian harmony to the region. In Chapter 4, I outlined in some detail how this European (and later American) influence blended with local performance practices to develop into some of the very songs that would help to harness the collective strength of an oppressed people. With few clear distinctions between religious, folk, and struggle songs, the repertoire of the liberation struggle drew from long-standing and deep connections between songs, community, and action.

However, while the subject of this book has been the songs and singers who have applied their culture and craft within the AIDS epidemic, and despite South Africa's rich performance cultures being fundamental to the arts-based interventions discussed in these pages, I have gone to some lengths to clearly articulate that musical effervescence is not an exclusively African phenomenon, it is a human one. In spite of its undeniable roots in Durkheim's ([1912] 2008) collective effervescence, a theory that was developed in response to late nineteenth and early twentieth-century analyses of indigenous Australian rituals (with all the preconceived colonial biases one might expect from such a time), musical effervescence highlights our common need for shared musical expression and experience. While universally applicable conceptions of music may be imprecise and ill-defined, the propensity for humans to move to and be moved by music (whatever it may sound like to different ears across cultures) is considerably less so. Throughout the analyses that followed my many observations and interactions during my time in South Africa, these concepts were crucial to understanding the ability of songs and singing to animate people and motivate desire for action that fundamentally influenced the course of the crisis.

Despite these insights, however, any book worth reading must be honest about what it is and is not able to achieve. My own work is, of course, no different and requires acknowledgment of its limitations. The first is that by balancing the broad with the specific, the general with the individual, some of the voices of those living with HIV have been lost. The writing in this book is equal parts historical ethnography and situated ethnography. As such, it has at times necessarily meandered around the conceptual edges of the kind of deeply embedded ethnographic approach that has become the modus operandi for most ethnomusicologists and anthropologists. While I have made every effort to ensure that individual voices and experiences are represented in these pages and have conducted considerable fieldwork in South Africa, the breadth of scope in this work—both geographically and conceptually—has limited the depth into which I may delve regarding any one particular organization, group, or community.

Secondly, this book cannot be understood as an exhaustive exploration of all musical approaches to the HIV/AIDS epidemic in South Africa. I have attempted to draw from a range of sources and artistic outputs, but there are, of course, omissions. These include songs by local artists and musicians that have specifically addressed HIV/AIDS (aside from those who were involved in 46664), practices that utilize songs within sangoma (traditional healer) medicinal practices, faith-based organizations, NGOs that have adopted song as a means of health communication (aside from the "ZAZI" music video), and local community music-making as social expression of disease.

Finally, while this book is concerned with songs and singing, it is important to note that there is a vast array of initiatives that fall outside the scope of these pages that employ the performing and creative arts for improved health and social outcomes around HIV/AIDS in South Africa. These include, but are not limited to, body mapping events popularized by the TAC, dance programs that draw from traditional cultural performance practices such as Nelisiwe Xaba's *Uncles and Angeles*, and the numerous forms of applied theater intervention performed by organizations such as Themba Interactive, DramAide, and Drama for Life.

Mirrors and Hammers: Songs in a Shifting Crisis

The HIV/AIDS crisis in South Africa has changed significantly since the early years of the epidemic. Since the early 2000s, substantial advances have been made in access to ARV medication—due in no small part to the efforts of the TAC—reducing stigma and blame, increasing AIDS awareness, and encouraging open discussion about the disease. Approaches to the epidemic have also changed. The once blunt message of "AIDS kills," deemed necessary throughout Africa in the early years of the continent's sub-Saharan crisis (van Buren 2011), has been steadily replaced with more nuanced understandings of the complex determinants of HIV transmission.

While it was formerly commonplace for priorities to be placed exclusively on biomedical interventions such as testing and pharmacological treatment, issues of structural violence and socioeconomic inequalities militated against health agency, exacerbating the effects of the epidemic among South Africa's underprivileged and vulnerable communities. Throughout this book, particularly in Chapter 2, I have attempted to highlight the connections between apartheid and AIDS, specifically noting the ways in which the ongoing legacies of White minority rule's socially engineered disenfranchisement provided the kindling from which the epidemic could rip through a nation.

In perhaps one of the more poignant excerpts from the literature on the topic, anthropologist Susan Levine (2012), during her fieldwork in the Cape Winelands township of Zwelethemba, notes that the local cemetery has expanded dramatically since the late 1990s. She describes the number of small wooden crosses that uniformly mark the resting places of recent AIDS victims and how they contrast with the more ornate and decorated apartheid-era graves.

In Zwelethemba, a narrow asphalt road demarcates the older apartheid graves from those who died more recently from AIDS, but while discussing the cost of human life with Levine, former political activist Miriam Moleleki suggested the metaphor of an invisible bridge connecting the two: one built from structural inequalities, poverty, racial injustice, and "a continuum of suffering across the generations" (64).

As a result of changes in the narrative of the epidemic, four broad themes have emerged throughout my analyses of the ways in which songs and singing have been applied within it. This thematic material conceptually maps a shifting epidemic over a period of more than twenty years. The first theme grew out of the prevailing silence around HIV/AIDS at the outset of the nascent crisis. Much has been written about this phenomenon as it relates to public health in the country (see Grünkemeier 2013; McNeill 2011; Decoteau 2013). The flurry of scholarly activity focused on AIDS in South Africa in the late 2000s and early 2010s that followed Barz's seminal work *Singing for Life* (2006) largely revolved around this concept and the ways in which musical cultures hindered or exacerbated this hesitance to speak openly about the virus (see Barz and Cohen 2011; McNeill 2011). It would seem fitting then that music, by definition an auditory sensorial experience, could provide some means through which to break this silence. High-profile events involving international recording artists became a familiar sound of the sonic landscape both within and outside of South Africa. Drawing inspiration from the humanitarian projects of the 1980s, the 46664 benefit concerts and music video HIV/AIDS awareness campaigns (discussed in Chapters 1, 5, and 9) were some of the most conspicuous events and campaigns to be employed for the purpose of normalizing open discussion about the disease.

While the activities of the TAC also contributed significantly toward this effort, the organization has been analyzed most readily in this book with reference to the second major set of themes, those of advocacy, activism, and community mobilization. Drawing from the cultural importance of songs—largely within the repertoires associated with the still very recent anti-apartheid struggle—the TAC employed tactical social marketing to create associations between their cause and the struggle for human rights. Musical effervescence played important roles in community-level mobilization toward health activism, with street movements, protests, sit-ins, and pickets energized through the collective singing of both old liberation songs and newer musical contributions to the second struggle for the right to health and life. Collective singing of these songs was credited with not only providing community support within the movement but even sustaining the physical strength of bodies weakened by AIDS for the duration of the demonstrations and rallies.

The TAC is most famous for their relentless pursuit of a nationally available HIV treatment program, and this book has discussed at length their applications of what I have elsewhere called "reservoirs of emotional potential" (Walker 2018, 176) through culturally resonant songs. However, what is less publicized, despite their important role in the aforementioned campaign and many high-profile performances and collaborations, is the HIV-positive choir The Generics that formed within the TAC during its early years of development. This choir encompasses the third set of themes that emerged while writing this book, those of community therapy and psychosocial healing.

Singing together with others facilitated a collectivization of grief, in a similar fashion to the numerous community choirs, faith-based choirs, and other local groups that involved communal singing during the apartheid era. The synchronization into shared space and time facilitated through communal music-making engendered a form of musical effervescence that was able to temporarily lift singers out of their current situation and into a new reality of ideals, such as those described by Durkheim ([1912] 2008). Ideal realities in which access to treatment is readily available, health is renewed through ARV therapies, medication is available to all, and people living with HIV are treated with dignity and respect.

The timbre and rhetoric of the AIDS epidemic began to shift in the late 2000s toward the final themes discussed in this book, those of HIV/AIDS awareness and prevention. This was largely a result of the increasing availability of ARV medication in the national public health system. As veteran AIDS activist Mandla Majola suggested during one of our interviews, the TAC has largely shifted its focus toward prevention-related issues.

> TAC has changed over the years. There is less urgency now. You must understand something: we were fighting for our lives and the lives of everyone who was living with HIV. In many ways that's still what TAC does today, but it's become more involved in prevention rather than the urgent need for ARV medication. People come to us because they want to help their community, so we offer to educate them on a specific issue so that the songs they sing and poems they perform will have accurate health information. They can become bridges between TAC and their community. Songs have been effective ways of doing that. In our own small way, we have used song to create awareness, to share pain, we have used song

> to vent out our anger, we have used song to educate people, for instance about HIV, or AIDS and rape. So, a song is not just a song, it's meaningless if it has no meaning. (Interview with Mandla Majola, June 2014)

This can also be seen in the number of prevention and awareness programs, such as the *Lucky, the Hero!* shows, that employ some of the more overt applications of musical effervescence to promote the reduction of AIDS-related stigma and encourage voluntary HIV testing.

The themes highlight the shifting roles that songs have played, and will likely continue to play, throughout the epidemic. I am reminded of an old adage, often attributed to German dramaturgist and playwright Bertolt Brecht, that art is not a mirror held up to reality, but a hammer through which to shape it. In the case of the songs of the South African AIDS crisis as discussed in this book, it would seem that Brecht was only half right. Songs did provide a hammer through which to shape the course of the epidemic, but those same songs also reflected the ever-changing social and political landscape of AIDS in South Africa.

This final chapter opened with an excerpt from a conversation that I had with Professor Jimmie Earl Perry in the summer of 2014. He spoke of the ways in which collective musical experiences influence individuals and groups both physically and emotionally, highlighting that an individual's background or socioeconomic status does not seem to hinder what appears to be a deeply embedded, culturally influenced, biological imperative to create connections through music. His words speak to the heart of this book. It has not been my intention to try to convince you that songs alone are necessarily the most effective methods for HIV awareness and prevention, activism and advocacy, or health and healing. Rather, there have been two main goals that I have sought to achieve. The first has been to highlight some of the various ways in which song has been employed within the HIV/AIDS epidemic; and how they have shaped and been shaped by the unfolding crisis. The second has been to furnish the reader with a framework—musical effervescence—through which to understand these seemingly disparate applications of song within the complex network of social, economic, cultural, and historical factors that have led to such a wealth of musical manifestations within the health crisis.

During my conversation with Mandla Majola mentioned earlier, he noted that, to him, a song is not just a song. While he was making reference to his experiences as an AIDS activist, his point is applicable to all the songs discussed in this book and elsewhere. For many people, music may seem like it has little practical use outside its commodified purpose as entertainment. But a song is more than just a song when it is used to express the intricacies and complexities of our humanity. It is more than just a song when it communicates simultaneously the profoundly social and deeply personal affective and emotive aspects of life, hope, death, loss, salvation, dignity, and triumph. It is more than just a song when its participatory and interpersonal qualities are fashioned into the connective tissues that bind together and facilitate the muscular political power of social movements. In these instances and beyond, the songs of the South African AIDS crisis were, and continue to be, so much more than just songs.

Note

1 The CPW is a government program designed to promote community cohesion. Particularly focused on women and young people, the program seeks to bring communities together for common purposes such as litter removal or small repair services, as well as providing an income for its members.

References

Adhikari, Mohamed. 2005. *Not White Enough, Not Black Enough: Racial Identity in the South African Coloured Community*. Athens, Cape Town: Ohio University Press; Double Storey.

Agawu, Kofi. 2003. *Representing African Music: Postcolonial Notes, Queries, Positions*. 1st ed. London: Routledge.

Ahmed, Sara. 2010. "Killing Joy: Feminism and the History of Happiness." *Signs: Journal of Women in Culture and Society* 35 (3): 571–94. https://doi.org/10.1086/648513.

Allen, Lara. 2003. "Commerce, Politics, and Musical Hybridity: Vocalizing Urban Black South African Identity during the 1950s." *Ethnomusicology* 47 (2): 228–49. https://doi.org/10.2307/3113919.

Alviso, Ric. 2011. "Tears Run Dry: Coping with AIDS through Music in Zimbabwe." In *The Culture of AIDS in Africa: Hope and Healing through Music*, edited by Gregory Barz and Judah Cohen, 56–62. New York: Oxford University Press. https://doi.org/10.1093/acprof:osobl/9780199744473.003.0004.

Anderson, Alison. 1997. *Media, Culture, and The Environment*. London: UCL.

Ansdell, Gary, Tia DeNora, and Sarah Ellen Wilson. 2016. *Musical Pathways in Recovery: Community Music Therapy and Mental Wellbeing*. London: Routledge.

Ansell, Gwen. 2005. *Soweto Blues: Jazz, Popular Music, and Politics in South Africa*. London: Bloomsbury Academic.

Armstrong, David, and Sherman Wilcox. 2007. *The Gestural Origin of Language*. Oxford: Oxford University Press.

Arnfred, Signe. 2004. "Rethinking Sexualities in Africa: Introduction." In *Re-Thinking Sexualities in Africa*, edited by Signe Arnfred, 7–34. Uppsala: Nordiska Afrikainstitutet.

Askew, Kelly, and Richard Wilks. 2002. "Introduction." In *The Anthropology of Media: A Reader*, edited by Kelly Askew, 1–13. Malden, MA & Oxford: Blackwell.

Athanasopoulos, George, Tuomas Eerola, Imre Lahdelma, and Maximos Kaliakatsos-Papakostas. 2021. "Harmonic Organisation Conveys Both Universal and Culture-Specific Cues for Emotional Expression in Music." *PLOS ONE* 16 (1): e0244964. https://doi.org/10.1371/journal.pone.0244964.

Aulette-Root, Anna, Floretta Boonzaier, and Judy Root Aulette. 2014. *South African Women Living with HIV: Global Lessons from Local Voices*. 1st ed. Bloomington: Indiana University Press.

Backer, Thomas, Everett Rogers, and Pradeep Sopory. 1992. *Designing Health Communication Campaigns: What Works?* Newbury Park, CA: Sage. https://doi.org/10.4135/9781483325521.

Badat, Saleem. 1999. *Black Student Politics: Higher Education and Apartheid from SASO to SANSCO, 1968–1990*. Pretoria: Human Sciences Research Council.

Baker, David, and Andy Bennett. 2022. "Good Citizenship, Telethon, and Benefit Concert: The Politics of the Achievable." In *Mixing Pop and Politics: Political Dimensions of Popular Music in the 21st Century*, edited by Catherine Hoad, Geoff Stahl, and Oli Wilson, 144–55. London: Routledge. https://doi.org/10.4324/9780429284526-13.

Baker, Peter. 2010. "From Apartheid to Neoliberalism: Health Equity in Post-Apartheid South Africa." *International Journal of Health Services* 40 (1): 79–95. https://doi.org/10.2190/hs.40.1.e.

Ballantine, Christopher. 1991. "Music and Emancipation: The Social Role of Black Jazz and Vaudeville in South Africa between the 1920s and the Early 1940s." *Journal of Southern African Studies* 17 (1): 129–52. https://doi.org/10.1080/03057079108708269.

Ballantine, Christopher. 1993. *Marabi Nights: Early South African Jazz and Vaudeville. Buch*. Johannesburg: Ravan Press.

Bandura, Albert. 1994. "Social Cognitive Theory and Exercise of Control over HIV Infection." In *Preventing AIDS: Theories and Methods of Behavioural Interventions*, edited by Ralph J. DiClemente and John L. Peterson, 1st ed., 25–59. New York: Springer.

Barton, Robert. 2006. "Primate Brain Evolution: Integrating Comparative, Neurophysiological, and Ethological Data." *Evolutionary Anthropology: Issues, News, and Reviews* 15 (6): 224–36. https://doi.org/10.1002/evan.20105.

Barz, Gregory. 2006. *Singing For Life HIV/AIDS and Music in Uganda*. 1st ed. New York: Routledge.

Barz, Gregory, and Judah Cohen. 2008. "Music and HIV/AIDS in Africa." In *The Garland Handbook of African Music*, edited by Ruth M Stone, 2nd ed., 148–59. New York: Routledge.

Barz, Gregory, and Judah Cohen. 2011. "Introduction: The Culture of AIDS: Hope and Healing Through the Arts in Africa." In *The Culture of AIDS in Africa: Hope and Healing Through Music and the Arts*, edited by Gregory Barz and Judah Cohen, 2–19. Oxford: Oxford University Press. https://doi.org/10.1093/acprof:osobl/9780199744473.001.0001.

Bateson, Gregory. 1972. *Steps to an Ecology of Mind: Collected Essays in Anthropology, Psychology, Evolution and Epistemology*. Chicago: University of Chicago.

Beck, Roger. 2000. *A History of South Africa*. Westport, Conn.: Greenwood Press.

Becker, John Joseph. 2011. "Rhythmic Entrainment and Evolution." In *Music, Science, and the Rhythmic Brain: Cultural and Clinical Implications*, edited by Jonathan Berger and Gabe Turow, 49–72. New York: Routledge.

Berger, Dorita, and Daniel Schneck. 2006. *The Music eEfect: Music Physiology and Clinical Applications*. London: Jessica Kingsley Publishers.

Berry, Gordon. 2007. "Television, Social Roles, and Marginality: Portrayals of the Past and Images for the Future." In *Children and Television: Fifty Years of Research*, edited by Norma Pecora, John Murray, and Ellen Ann Wartella, 85–108. London: Lawrence Erlbaum Associates.

Bhana, Deevia, and Rob Pattman. 2011. "Girls Want Money, Boys Want Virgins: The Materiality of Love Amongst South African Township Youth in the Context of HIV and AIDS." *Culture, Health & Sexuality* 13 (8): 961–72. https://doi.org/10.1080/13691058.2011.576770.

Biehl, João. 2004. "The Activist State." *Social Text* 22 (3): 105–32. https://doi.org/10.1215/01642472-22-3_80-105.

Biehl, João. 2005. *Vita: Life in a Zone of Social Abandonment*. Berkeley: University of California Press.

Black, Steven P. 2019. *Speech and Songs on the Margins of Global Health: Zulu Tradition, HIV Stigma, and AIDS Activism in South Africa*. New Jersey: Rutgers University Press.

Blacking, John, Reginald Byron, and Bruno Nettl. 1995. *Music, Culture, & Experience: Selected Papers of John Blacking*. Chicago: University of Chicago Press.

Blacking, John. 1974. *How Musical Is Man?* Seattle: University of Washington Press.

Blacking, John. 1985. "The Context of Venda Possession Music: Reflections on the Effectiveness of Symbols." *Yearbook for Traditional Music* 17: 64–87. https://doi.org/10.2307/768437.

Blacking, John. 1987. *A Commonsense View of All Music: Reflections on Percy Grainger's Contribution to Ethnomusicology and Music Education*. Cambridge: Cambridge University Press.

Blacking, John. 1969. "Songs, Dances, Mimes and Symbolism of Venda Girls' Initiation Schools: Part 4: The Great Domba Song." *African Studies* 28 (4): 215–66. https://doi.org/10.1080/00020186908707313.

Blacking, John. [1967] 1995. *Venda Children's Songs: A Study in Ethnomusicological Analysis*. Chicago: University of Chicago Press. Originally published in 1967 by Witwatersrand University Press.

Bleakley, Alan. 2013. "Towards a Critical Medical Humanities." In *Medicine, Health and the Arts: Approaches to the Medical Humanities*, edited by Victoria Bates, Alan Bleakley, and Sam Goodman, 17–26. London: Routledge.

Bleakley, Alan. 2015. *Medical Humanities and Medical Education: How the Medical Humanities Can Shape Better Doctors*. 1st ed. New York: Routledge.

Boonzaier, Floretta. 2005. "Woman Abuse in South Africa: A Brief Contextual Analysis." *Feminism & Psychology* 15 (1): 99–103. https://doi.org/10.1177/0959353505049711.

Bottomley, Edward-John. 2012. *Poor White*. 1st ed. Cape Town, South Africa: Tafelberg.

Bourgault, Louise Manon. 2003. *Playing for Life: Performance in Africa in the Age of AIDS*. Durham, N.C: Carolina Academic Press.

Bozzoli, Belinda. 2004. *Theatres of Struggle and the End of Apartheid*. Edinburgh: Edinburgh University Press.

Brehm, Jack. 1966. *A Theory of Psychological Reactance*. New York: Academic Press.

Brehm, Jack, and Sharon Brehm. 1981. *Psychological Reactance: A Theory of Freedom and Control*. New York: Academic Press.

Breitinger, Eckhard. 2011. "HIV/AIDS Poster Campaigns in Malawi." In *The Culture of AIDS in Africa: Hope and Healing Through Music and the Arts*, edited by Gregory Barz and Judah Cohen, 131–43. Oxford: Oxford University Press. https://doi.org/10.1093/acprof:osobl/9780199744473.003.0012.

Brown, Steven. 2000. "The 'Musilanguage' Model of Music Evolution." In *The Origins of Music*, edited by Nils L. Wallin, Björn Merker, and Steven Brown. MIT Press. Cambridge, MA, USA. https://doi.org/10.7551/mitpress/5190.003.0022.

Brown, Steven. 2017. "A Joint Prosodic Origin of Language and Music." *Frontiers in Psychology* 8: 1894. https://doi.org/10.3389/fpsyg.2017.01894.

Bruinders, Sylvia. 2010. "Parading Respectability: The Christmas Bands Movement in the Western Cape, South Africa and the Constitution of Subjectivity." *African Music: Journal of the International Library of African Music* 8 (4): 69–83. https://doi.org/10.21504/amj.v8i4.1867.

Bryant, Alfred. 1949. *The Zulu People, as They Were Before the White Man Came*. Pietermaritzburg: Shuter and Shooter.

Calhoun-Brown, Allison. 2000. "Upon This Rock: The Black Church, Nonviolence, and the Civil Rights Movement." *PS: Political Science & Politics* 33 (2): 169–74. https://doi.org/10.2307/420886.

Campbell, Polly, Alexander Ophir, and Steven Phelps. 2009. "Central Vasopressin and Oxytocin Receptor Distributions in Two Species of Singing Mice." *Journal of Comparative Neurology* 516 (4): 321–33. https://doi.org/10.1002/cne.22116.

Cavicchi, Daniel. 2002. "From the Bottom up: Thinking about Tia DeNora's Music in Everyday Life." *Action, Criticism, and Theory for Music Education* 1 (2): 2–15.

Chalmers, John. 1878. *Tiyo Soga: A Page of South Africa Missionary Work*. Edinburgh: A. Elliot.

Changizi, Mark. 2011. *Harnessed: How Language and Music Mimicked Nature and Transformed Ape to Man*. Dallas, Tex: BenBella Books.

Cherry, Janet. 2015. "Emzabalazweni: Singing the Language of the Struggle, Past and Present." In *Singing, Speaking and Writing Politics: South African Political Discourses*, edited by Mirjana N Dedaić, 221–46. Amsterdam: John Benjamins Publishing. https://doi.org/10.1075/dapsac.65.10che.

Chigwedere, Pride, George Seage, Sofia Gruskin, Tun-Hou Lee, and Morgan Essex. 2008. "Estimating the Lost Benefits of Antiretroviral Drug Use in South Africa."

JAIDS Journal of Acquired Immune Deficiency Syndromes 49 (4): 410–15. https://doi.org/10.1097/qai.0b013e31818a6cd5.

Chikowero, Mhoze. 2015. *African Music, Power, and Being in Colonial Zimbabwe.* Bloomington: Indiana University Press.

Chinyowa, Kennedy. 2009. "Theatrical Performance as Technology: The Case of Drama in Aids Education (DramAidE) in South Africa." *Studies in Theatre and Performance* 29 (1): 33–52. https://doi.org/10.1386/stap.29.1.33_1.

Clare, Amy, and Paul Camic. 2019. "Live and Recorded Group Music Interventions with Active Participation for People with Dementias: A Systematic Review." *Arts & Health* 12 (3): 197–220. https://doi.org/10.1080/17533015.2019.1675732.

Clayton, Martin, Rebecca Sager, and Udo Will. 2004. "In Time with The Music: The Concept of Entrainment and Its Significance for Ethnomusicology." *European Meetings in Ethnomusicology* 1 (11): 3–142.

Clee, Mona, and Robert Wicklund. 1980. "Consumer Behavior and Psychological Reactance." *Journal of Consumer Research* 6 (4): 389. https://doi.org/10.1086/208782.

Cole, Abimbola. 2011. "Contemporary Uses of the Musical Arts in Botswana's HIV/AIDS Health Education Initiatives: The Case of the Radio Serial Drama Makgabaneng." In *The Culture of AIDS in Africa: Hope and Healing Through Music and the Arts*, edited by Gregory Barz and Judah Cohen, 144–57. Oxford: Oxford University Press. https://doi.org/10.1093/acprof:osobl/9780199744473.003.0013.

Collins, Randall. 2004. *Interaction Ritual Chains.* Princeton, N.J: Princeton University Press.

"Community Media Trust AIDS Archive." n.d. Ibali - Digital Collections UCT. CC-BY-NC 4.0. Accessed July 20, 2024. https://ibali.uct.ac.za/s/ibali/page/welcome.

Confucius. 2012. "The Musical Records." In *Contemporary Chinese Aesthetics*, edited by Zhu Liyuan and Gene Blocker. New York: Peter Lang Publishing Inc. https://doi.org/10.3726/978-1-4539-0999-7.

Conway, Daniel. 2007. "The Masculine State in Crisis: State Response to War Resistance in Apartheid South Africa." *Men and Masculinities* 10 (4): 422–39. https://doi.org/10.1177/1097184x07306742.

Condillac, Étienne. [1746] 1971. *An Essay on the Origin of Human Knowledge.* Translated by R. G. Weyant, 1756. Gainesville, FL: Scholars' Facsimiles and Reprints.

Cook, Nicholas. 1994. "Music and Meaning in the Commercials." *Popular Music* 13 (1): 27–40. https://doi.org/10.1017/s0261143000006826.

Cook, Nicholas. 1998. *Music: A Very Short Introduction.* Oxford: Oxford University Press.

Cook, Nicholas. 2001. "Theorizing Musical Meaning." *Music Theory Spectrum* 23 (2): 170–95. https://doi.org/10.1525/mts.2001.23.2.170.

Cooper, Andrew. 2008. "Beyond One Image Fits All: Bono and the Complexity of Celebrity Diplomacy." *Global Governance: A Review of Multilateralism and*

International Organizations 14 (3): 265–72. https://doi.org/10.1163/19426720-01403002.

Coplan, David. 1985. *In Township Tonight!: South Africa's Black City Music and Theatre.* Addison-Wesley Longman Ltd. London, UK.

Cousins, Laura. 2009. "Modelling Cross-Gender and Sexual Relations: Exploring the Soul Buddyz Edutainment Initiative in South Africa." *ISS Working Paper Series / General Series*, 1765018728, 465: 1–63. https://hdl.handle.net/1765/18728.

Crossley, Nick. 2020. *Connecting Sounds: The Social Life of Music.* Manchester: Manchester University Press.

Cummins, Fred. 2009. "Rhythm as Entrainment: The Case of Synchronous Speech." *Journal of Phonetics* 37 (1): 16–28. https://doi.org/10.1016/j.wocn.2008.08.003.

Dargie, David. 1997. "Christian Music Among South Africans." In *Christianity in South Africa: A Political, Social and Cultural History*, edited by Richard Elphick and Rodney Davenport, 317–19. Berkley: University of California Press.

Darwin, Charles. 1871. *The Descent of Man, and Selection in Relation to Sex.* 1st ed., Vol. 1. New York: Rand McNally.

Davidson, Jane, and Sandra Garrido. 2016. *Music and Mourning.* London: Taylor & Francis.

Davis, Heloïse Victoria. 2012. "Theatre as Intervention Tool in HIV/AIDS Education with Specific Reference to 'Lucky, the Hero!'" Master's thesis, Stellenbosch University. http://hdl.handle.net/10019.1/20247.

Decoteau, Claire Laurier. 2008. "The Bio-Politics of HIV/AIDS in Post-Apartheid South Africa." Doctoral thesis, University of Michigan. https://deepblue.lib.umich.edu/handle/2027.42/61711.

Decoteau, Claire Laurier. 2013. *Ancestors and Antiretrovirals: The Biopolitics of HIV/AIDS in Post-Apartheid South Africa.* Chicago and London: The University of Chicago Press.

Delius, Peter, and Clive Glaser. 2002. "Sexual Socialisation in South Africa: A Historical Perspective." *African Studies* 61 (1): 27–54. https://doi.org/10.1080/00020180220140064.

DeNora, Tia. 2000. *Music in Everyday Life.* Cambridge: Cambridge University Press.

DeNora, Tia. 2013. *Music Asylums: Wellbeing Through Music in Everyday Life.* Surrey: Ashgate.

Denselow, Robin. 1989. *When the Music's over: The Story of Political Pop.* London: Faber & Faber.

Diener, Ed, Rob Lusk, Darlene DeFour, and Robert Flax. 1980. "Deindividuation: Effects of Group Size, Density, Number of Observers, and Group Member Similarity on Self-Consciousness and Disinhibited Behavior." *Journal of Personality and Social Psychology* 39 (3): 449–59. https://doi.org/10.1037/0022-3514.39.3.449.

Dieter, Heribert, and Rajiv Kumar. 2008. "The Downside of Celebrity Diplomacy: The Neglected Complexity of Development." *Global Governance: A Review of*

Multilateralism and International Organizations 14 (3): 259–64. https://doi.org/10.1163/19426720-01403001.

Díaz, Juan Diego. 2021. *Africanness in Action: Essentialism and Musical Imaginations of Africa in Brazil*. New York: Oxford University Press.

Donovan, Robert, and Nadine Henley. 2010. *Principles and Practice of Social Marketing: An International Perspective*. Cambridge: Cambridge University Press.

Dooling, Wayne. 2007. *Slavery, Emancipation and Colonial Rule in South Africa*. Athens: Ohio University Press.

Drewett, Michael. 2007. "'Stop This Filth': The Censorship of Roger Lucey's Music in Apartheid South Africa." *South African Music Studies* 25 (1): 53–71. https://doi.org/10.4314/samus.v25i1.6403.

Drewett, Michael. 2008. "Developing a Retro Brand Community: Re-releasing and Marketing Anti-Apartheid Protest Music in Post-Apartheid South Africa.". *Consumption Markets and Culture* 11 (4): 287–305. https://doi.org/10.1080/10253860802391292.

du Toit, Louise. 2014. "Shifting Meanings of Postconflict Sexual Violence in South Africa." *Signs: Journal of Women in Culture and Society* 40 (1): 101–23. https://doi.org/10.1086/676895.

Dunbar, Robin. 1996. *Grooming, Gossip and the Evolution of Language*. London: Faber & Faber.

Dunbar, Robin. 2003. "The Social Brain: Mind, Language, and Society in Evolutionary Perspective." *Annual Review of Anthropology* 32 (1): 163–81. https://doi.org/10.1146/annurev.anthro.32.061002.093158.

Dunbar, Robin. 2012. "On the Evolutionary Function of Song and Dance." In *Music, Language, and Human Evolution*, edited by Nicholas Bannan, 201–14. Oxford: Oxford University Press. https://doi.org/10.1093/acprof:osobl/9780199227341.003.0008.

Dunbar, Robin. 2017. "Group Size, Vocal Grooming and the Origins of Language." *Psychonomic Bulletin & Review* 24 (1): 209–12. https://doi.org/10.3758/s13423-016-1122-6.

Dunbar, Robin, and Susanne Shultz. 2007. "Understanding Primate Brain Evolution." *Philosophical Transactions of the Royal Society B: Biological Sciences* 362 (1480): 649–58. https://doi.org/10.1098/rstb.2006.2001.

Durkheim, Émile. [1912] 2008. *The Elementary Forms of the Religious Life*. Translated by Joseph Ward Swain. Mineola, NY: Dover Publications.

Eck, Douglas, Michael Gasser, and Robert Port. 2000. "Dynamics and Embodiment in Beat Induction." *Rhythm Perception and Production*, 157–70.

Eller-Isaacs, Jonah. 2011. "Singing in the Shadow of Death: African Musicians Respond to a Pandemic with Songs of Sorrow, Resistance, Advocacy, and Hope." In *The Culture of AIDS in Africa: Hope and Healing through Music*, edited by Gregory Barz and Judah Cohen, 63–9. Oxford: Oxford University Press. https://doi.org/10.1093/acprof:osobl/9780199744473.003.0005.

Elmashhara, Maher Georges, and Ana Maria Soares. 2020. "The Influence of Atmospherics General Interior Variables on Shoppers' Emotions and Behavior." *The International Review of Retail, Distribution and Consumer Research* 30 (4): 437–59. https://doi.org/10.1080/09593969.2020.1724556.

Erasmus, Zimitri. 2001. *Coloured by History, Shaped by Place: New Perspectives on Coloured Identities in Cape Town*. Cape Town: Kwela Books.

Erlmann, Veit. 1990. "Migration and Performance: Zulu Migrant Workers' Isicathamiya Performance in South Africa, 1890–1950." *Ethnomusicology* 34 (2): 199. https://doi.org/10.2307/851683.

Erlmann, Veit. 1991. *African Stars: Studies in Black South African Performance*. Chicago: University of Chicago Press.

Erlmann, Veit. 1996. *Nightsong: Performance, Power, and Practice in South Africa*. Chicago: University of Chicago Press.

Erlmann, Veit. 1999. *Music, Modernity, and the Global Imagination: South Africa and the West*. New York: Oxford Scholarship Online.

Evans, Martha. 2014. *Broadcasting the End of Apartheid: Live Television and the Birth of the New South Africa*. London: I.B. Tauris.

Faria, Nuno, Andrew Rambaut, Marc A. Suchard, Guy Baele, Trevor Bedford, Melissa J. Ward, Andrew J. Tatem, et al. 2014. "HIV Epidemiology: The Early Spread and Epidemic Ignition of HIV-1 in Human Populations." *Science* 346 (6205): 56–61. https://doi.org/10.1126/science.1256739.

Farmer, Paul. 1992. *AIDS and Accusation: Haiti and the Geography of Blame*. Berkeley: University of California Press.

Farmer, Paul. 1999. *Infections and Inequalities: The Modern Plagues*. Berkeley, CA: University of California.

Farmer, Paul. 2004. "An Anthropology of Structural Violence." *Current Anthropology* 45 (3): 305–25. https://doi.org/10.1086/382250.

Farmer, Paul. 2005. *Pathologies of Power Health, Human Rights, and the New War on the Poor*. Berkeley, CA: University of California Press.

Farmer, Paul. 2009. "On Suffering and Structural Violence: A View from Below." *Race/Ethnicity: Multidisciplinary Global Contexts* 3 (1): 11–28. https://www.jstor.org/stable/25595022.

Fassin, Didier. 2007. *When Bodies Remember: Experiences and Politics of AIDS in South Africa*. Los Angeles: Univ. of California Press.

Feinstein, Charles Hilliard. 2005. *An Economic History of South Africa: Conquest, Discrimination and Development*. Cambridge: Cambridge University Press.

Feld, Steven. 1988. "Aesthetics as Iconicity of Style, or 'Lift-up-over Sounding': Getting into the Kaluli Groove." *Yearbook for Traditional Music* 20: 74–113. https://doi.org/10.2307/768167.

Fischer-Lichte, Erika. 2007. *Theatre, Sacrifice, Ritual Exploring Forms of Political Theatre*. Florence: Taylor and Francis.

Fleagle, John, Zelalem Assefa, Francis Brown, and John Shea. 2008. "Paleoanthropology of the Kibish Formation, Southern Ethiopia: Introduction." *Journal of Human Evolution* 55 (3): 360–65. https://doi.org/10.1016/j.jhevol.2008.05.007.

Floody, Owen, Tim Cooper, and Elliott Albers. 1998. "Injection of Oxytocin into the Medial Preoptic–Anterior Hypothalamus Increases Ultrasound Production by Female Hamsters." *Peptides* 19 (5): 833–39. https://doi.org/10.1016/s0196-9781(98)00029-1.

Fordham, Graham. 2015. *HIV/AIDS and the Social Consequences of Untamed Biomedicine: Anthropological Complicities*. London: Routledge.

Fourie, Pieter, and Melissa Meyer. 2010. *The Politics of AIDS Denialism: South Africa's Failure to Respond*. Abingdon, Oxon: Routledge.

Friedson, Steven. 1996. *Dancing Prophets: Musical Experience in Tumbuka Healing*. Chicago: University of Chicago Press.

Gamson, Josh. 1989. "Silence, Death, and the Invisible Enemy: AIDS Activism and Social Movement 'Newness.'" *Social Problems* 36 (4): 351–67. https://doi.org/10.2307/800820.

Garofalo, Reebee. 2005. "Who Is the World?: Reflections on Music and Politics Twenty Years after Live Aid." *Journal of Popular Music Studies* 17 (3): 324–44. https://doi.org/10.1111/j.1524-2226.2005.00048.x.

Gaulier, Armelle, and Denis Martin. 2017. *Cape Town Harmonies: Memory, Humour and Resilience*. Cape Town: African Minds.

Geffen, Nathan. 2010. *Debunking Delusions: The Inside Story of the Treatment Action Campaign*. Auckland Park: Jacana Media.

Gilbert, Shirli. 2005. "Popular Song, Gender Equality and the Arti-Apartheid Struggle." In *Gender and Sexuality in South African Music*, edited by Chris Walton and Stephanus Muller, 11–18. Stellenbosch: African SUN Media.

Gilbert, Shirli. 2007. "Singing against Apartheid: ANC Cultural Groups and the International Anti-Apartheid Struggle." *Journal of Southern African Studies* 33 (2): 421–41. https://doi.org/10.1080/03057070701292848.

Gillespie-Lynch, Kristen, Patricia Marks Greenfield, Yuntian Feng, Sue Savage-Rumbaugh, and Heidi. Lyn. 2013. "A Cross-Species Study of Gesture and Its Role in Symbolic Development: Implications for the Gestural Theory of Language Evolution." *Frontiers in Psychology* 4. https://doi.org/10.3389/fpsyg.2013.00160.

Gorn, Gerald. 1982. "The Effects of Music in Advertising on Choice Behavior: A Classical Conditioning Approach." *Journal of Marketing* 46 (1): 94–101. https://doi.org/10.2307/1251163.

Grahn, Jessica, Molly J. Henry, and J. Devin McAuley. 2011. "FMRI Investigation of Cross-Modal Interactions in Beat Perception: Audition Primes Vision, but Not Vice Versa." *NeuroImage* 54 (2): 1231–43. https://doi.org/10.1016/j.neuroimage.2010.09.033.

Grape, Christina, Maria Sandgren, Lars-Olof Hansson, Mats Ericson, and Töres Theorell. 2003. "Does Singing Promote Well-Being?: An Empirical Study of Professional and Amateur Singers during a Singing Lesson." *Integrative Physiological & Behavioral Science* 38 (1): 65–74. https://doi.org/10.1007/bf02734261.

Gray, Anne-Marie. 2004. "The Liberation Songs: An Important Voice of Black South Africans from 1912 to 1994." Journal of Education 33 (1): 85–102.

Grebe, Eduard. 2011. "The Treatment Action Campaign's Struggle for AIDS Treatment in South Africa: Coalition-Building Through Networks." *Journal of Southern African Studies* 37 (4): 849–68. https://doi.org/10.1080/03057070.2011.608271.

Greenberg, Bradley, Charles Salmon, Dhaval Patel, Vicki Beck, and Galen Cole. 2004. "Evolution of an E-E Research Agenda." In *Entertainment-Education and Social Change History, Research, and Practice*, edited by Arvind Singhal, Michael Cody, Everett Rogers, and Miguel Sabido, 1st ed. New Jersey: Lawrence Erlbaum Associates.

Gregg, Melissa, and Gregory Seigworth. 2010. *The Affect Theory Reader*. Durham, NC: Duke University Press.

Grünkemeier, Ellen. 2013. *Breaking the Silence: South African Representations of HIV*. New York: Boydell & Brewer.

Guccione, Bob. 1986. "Who's Who, What's What, and Why." *Spin Magazine*, July.

Gunner, Liz. 2003. "'Those Dying Generations at Their Song': Singing of Life, Death and Aids in Contemporary KwaZulu-Natal." *English Studies in Africa* 46 (2): 41–53. https://doi.org/10.1080/00138390308691010.

Hall, Edward Twitchell. 1976. *Beyond Culture*. New York: Anchor Books.

Hall, Stuart. 1973. "Encoding and Decoding in the Television Discourse." *CCCS Selected Working Papers* 2: 386–98.

Hall, Stuart. 1980. "Cultural Studies: Two Paradigms." *Media, Culture & Society* 2 (1): 57–72. https://doi.org/10.1177/016344378000200106.

Harrison, Scott, Marie Cooke, Wendy Moyle, David Shum, and Jenny Elaine Murfield. 2010. "Development of a Music Intervention Protocol and Its Effect on Participant Engagement: Experiences from a Randomised Controlled Trial with Older People with Dementia." *Arts & Health* 2 (2): 125–39. https://doi.org/10.1080/17533015.2010.490839.

Harvey, Alan. 2017. "Music, Altruism, and Social Cooperation." In *Music, Evolution, and the Harmony of Souls*, 144–60. Oxford: Oxford University Press. https://doi.org/10.1093/acprof:oso/9780198786856.003.0005.

Hatten, Robert. 2004. *Interpreting Musical Gestures, Topics, and Tropes: Mozart, Beethoven, Schubert*. Bloomington, IN: Indiana University Press. https://doi.org/10.2307/j.ctt2005zts.

Henderson, Patricia. 2011. *AIDS, Intimacy and Care in Rural KwaZulu-Natal: A Kinship of Bones*. Amsterdam: Amsterdam University Press.

Hesmondhalgh, David. 2013. *Why Music Matters*. Chichester, West Sussex: John Wiley & Sons Ltd.

Higginson, John. 2014. *Collective Violence and the Agrarian Origins of South African Apartheid, 1900–48*. Cambridge: Cambridge University Press.

Hinson, Glenn. 2000. *Fire in My Bones: Transcendence and the Holy Spirit in African American Gospel*. Philadelphia: University of Pennsylvania Press.

Hirsch, Lee, dir. 2002. *Amandla!: A Revolution in Four-Part Harmony*. Produced by Sherry Simpson Dean and Desiree Markgraaf. South Africa: ATO Pictures. New York.

Hodes, Rebecca. 2011. "'We Are the Loudmouthed HIV-Positive People': 'Siyayinqoba/ Beat It!' On South African Television." In *The Culture of AIDS in Africa: Hope and Healing Through Music*, edited by Gregory Barz and Judah Cohen, 158–79. New York: Oxford University Press. https://doi.org/10.1093/acprof:osobl/9780199744473.003.0014.

Home, Felicity June. 2005. "Yesterday, AIDS and Structural Violence in South Africa." *Communication* 31 (2): 172–97. https://doi.org/10.1080/02500160508538001.

Hongoro, Charles, Getnet Tadele, and Helmut Kloos. 2013. "HIV/AIDS and the Mining and Commercial Agricultural Sectors in Southern Africa." In *Vulnerabilities, Impacts, and Responses to HIV/AIDS in Sub-Saharan Africa*, edited by Getnet Tadele and Helmut Kloos, 127–42. London: Palgrave Macmillan. https://doi.org/10.1057/9781137009951_7.

Honing, Henkjan, Olivia Ladinig, Gábor Háden, and István Winkler. 2009. "Is Beat Induction Innate or Learned?" *Annals of the New York Academy of Sciences* 1169 (1): 93–6. https://doi.org/10.1111/j.1749-6632.2009.04761.x.

Howes, David, and Constance Classen. 2014. *Ways of Sensing: Understanding the Senses in Society*. New York: Routledge.

Huliaras, Asteris, and Nikolaos Tzifakis. 2012. "The Fallacy of the Autonomous Celebrity Activist in International Politics: George Clooney and Mia Farrow in Darfur." *Cambridge Review of International Affairs* 25 (3): 417–31. https://doi.org/10.1080/09557571.2012.710591.

Hunt, Kevin. 1994. "The Evolution of Human Bipedality: Ecology and Functional Morphology." *Journal of Human Evolution* 26 (3): 183–202. https://doi.org/10.1006/jhev.1994.1011.

Hunter, Mark. 2002. "The Materiality of Everyday Sex: Thinking beyond 'Prostitution.'" *African Studies* 61 (1): 99–120. https://doi.org/10.1080/00020180220140091.

Hunter, Mark. 2007. "The Changing Political Economy of Sex in South Africa: The Significance of Unemployment and Inequalities to the Scale of the AIDS Pandemic." *Social Science & Medicine* 64 (3): 689–700. https://doi.org/10.1016/j.socscimed.2006.09.015.

Hunter, Mark. 2010. *Love in the Time of AIDS: Inequality, Gender, and Rights in South Africa*. Bloomington: Indiana University Press.

Hurley, Erin, and Sara Warner. 2012. "Special Section: 'Affect/Performance/Politics.'" *Journal of Dramatic Theory and Criticism* 26 (2): 99–107. https://doi.org/10.1353/dtc.2012.0000.

Huron, David. 1989. "Music in Advertising: An Analytic Paradigm." *The Musical Quarterly* 73 (4): 557–74. https://doi.org/10.1093/mq/73.4.557.

Impey, Angela. 2008. "Popular Music in Africa." In *The Garland Handbook of African Music.* 2nd ed., edited by Ruth M. Stone, 124–47. New York: Routledge.

Jablonka, Eva, Simona Ginsburg, and Daniel Dor. 2012. "The Co-Evolution of Language and Emotions." *Philosophical Transactions of the Royal Society B: Biological Sciences* 367 (1599): 2152–9. https://doi.org/10.1098/rstb.2012.0117.

Jack, Max. 2021. "The Crowd in Flux: Atmosphere and the Governance of Public Affects at FC Union Berlin." *Ethnomusicology* 65 (3): 497–518. https://doi.org/10.5406/ethnomusicology.65.3.0497.

Jaffe-Berg, Erith. 2001. "Forays into Grammelot: The Language of Nonsense." *Journal of Dramatic Theory and Criticism* 15 (2): 3–16. https://doi.org/https://doi.org/10.17161/jdtc.v0i2.3364.

Jansen, Jonathan. 2017. *As by Fire: The End of the South African University.* Cape Town: Tafelberg.

Jeeves, Alan. 1985. *Migrant Labour in South Africa's Mining Economy: Struggle for the Gold Mines' Labour Supply 1890–1920.* Kingston: McGill-Queen's University Press.

Jeffreys, Elaine, and Paul Allatson. 2015. *Celebrity Philanthropy.* Bristol: Intellect.

Jewkes, Rachel, Kristin Dunkle, Mzikazi Nduna, and Nwabisa Shai. 2010. "Intimate Partner Violence, Relationship Power Inequity, and Incidence of HIV Infection in Young Women in South Africa: A Cohort Study." *The Lancet* 376 (9734): 41–48. https://doi.org/10.1016/s0140-6736(10)60548-x.

Johnson, Caroline, and Corey Wagner. 2011. "I've Got You under My Skin: Differential Implicit and Explicit Responses to Music in Advertising." *American Academy of Advertising Conference Proceedings*, 123–31.

Kalichman, Seth, Leickness Chisamu Simbayi, Redwaan Vermaak, Sean Jooste, and Demetria Cain. 2008. "HIV/AIDS Risks among Men and Women Who Drink at Informal Alcohol Serving Establishments (Shebeens) in Cape Town, South Africa." *Prevention Science* 9 (1): 55–62. https://doi.org/10.1007/s11121-008-0085-x.

Kallen, Stuart. 2011. *Open the Jail Doors -- We Want to Enter: The Defiance Campaign against Apartheid Laws, South Africa, 1952.* Minneapolis: Twenty-First Century Books.

Kandirikirira, Niki. 2002. "Deconstructing Domination: Gender Disempowerment and the Legacy of Colonialism and Apartheid in Omaheke, Namibia." In *Masculinities Matter: Men, Gender and Development*, edited by Frances Cleaver, 112–37. London: Zed Books Ltd.

Kapoor, Ilan. 2013. *Celebrity Humanitarianism: The Ideology of Global Charity.* New York: Routledge.

Karim, Quarraisha Abdool. 2010. "Heterosexual Transmission of HIV – the Importance of a Gendered Perspective in HIV Prevention." In *HIV/AIDS in South Africa*, edited by S. S. Abdool Karim and Q. Abdool Karim, 285–304. Cambridge: Cambridge University Press.

Kauffman, Kyle Dean, and David Lindauer, eds. 2004. *AIDS and South Africa: The Social Expression of a Pandemic*. New York: Palgrave Macmillan.

Keil, Charles, and Steven Feld. 1994. *Music Grooves: Essays and Dialogues*. Chicago: University of Chicago Press.

Kertzer, David I. 1988. *Ritual, Politics, and Power*. New Haven: London: Yale University Press.

Kivnick, Helen. 1990. *Where Is the Way: Song and Struggle in South Africa*. New York: Penguin Books.

Koen, Benjamin. 2009. *Beyond the Rooftop of the World*. Oxford: Oxford University Press.

Koen, Benjamin D., Jacqueline Lloyd, Gregory Barz, and Karen Brummel-Smith. 2008. *The Oxford Handbook of Medical Ethnomusicology*. New York: Oxford University Press.

Kooijman, Jaap. 2008. *Fabricating the Absolute Fake: America in Contemporary Pop Culture*. Amsterdam: Amsterdam University Press.

Kritzinger, Karin. 2013. "The Struggle for Justice in South Africa (1986–1990): The Participation of the Dutch Reformed Mission Church and the Dutch Reformed Church." In *Reformed Churches in South Africa and the Struggle for Justice: Remembering 1960–1990*, edited by Marry-Anne Plaatjies-Van Huffel and Robert Vosloo, 92–117. Stellenbosch: Sun Press.

Krueger, Joel. 2014. "Affordances and the Musically Extended Mind." *Frontiers in Psychology* 4. https://doi.org/10.3389/fpsyg.2013.01003.

Large, Edward, and John Kolen. 1994. "Resonance and the Perception of Musical Meter." *Connection Science* 6 (2–3): 177–208. https://doi.org/10.1080/09540099408915723.

Larsson, Matz, Joachim Richter, and Andrea Ravignani. 2019. "Bipedal Steps in the Development of Rhythmic Behavior in Humans." *Music & Science* 2 (January). https://doi.org/10.1177/2059204319892617.

Le Bon, Gustave. [1895] 2009. *The Crowd: A Study of the Popular Mind*. Auckland: The Floating Press.

Lee, Nancy C. 2010. *Lyrics of Lament: From Tragedy to Transformation*. Minneapolis: Fortress Press.

Leman, Marc, Dirk Moelants, Matthias Varewyck, Frederik Styns, Leon van Noorden, and Jean-Pierre Martens. 2013. "Activating and Relaxing Music Entrains the Speed of Beat Synchronized Walking." *PLOS ONE* 8 (7): e67932. https://doi.org/10.1371/journal.pone.0067932.

Lemieux, Anthony, Jeffrey Fisher, and Felicia Pratto. 2008. "A Music-Based HIV Prevention Intervention for Urban Adolescents." *Health Psychology* 27 (3): 349–57. https://doi.org/10.1037/0278-6133.27.3.349.

Lesch, Elmien, and Lou-Marie Kruger. 2004. "Reflections on the Sexual Agency of Young Women in a Low-Income Rural South African Community." *South African Journal of Psychology* 34 (3): 464–86. https://doi.org/10.1177/008124630403400308.

Levine, Susan, and Fiona Ross. 2002. "Perceptions of and Attitudes to HIV/AIDS among Young Adults in Cape Town." *Social Dynamics* 28 (1): 89–108. https://doi.org/10.1080/02533950208458724.

Levine, Susan. 2007. "Documentary Film Matters: The Steps for the Future Media Advocacy Project in Southern Africa." *Critical Arts* 21 (2): 234–49. https://doi.org/10.1080/02560040701810024.

Levine, Susan. 2012. "Testing Knowledge: Legitimacy, Healing and Medicine in South Africa." In *Medicine and the Politics of Knowledge*, 55–78. Cape Town: HSRC Press.

Lewis, Jack, and Lucilla Blankenberg. 2011. *Taking Haart*. Cape Town: Community Media Trust.

Lindfors, Bernth. 2021. "The Rise and Fall of Mbongeni Ngema: The AIDS Play." *In South African Theatre as/and Intervention*, edited by Marcia Blumberg and Dennis Walder, 181–91. Leiden: Brill.

Ludden, David. 2016. *The Psychology of Language: An Integrated Approach*. London: SAGE.

Lurie, Mark. 2010. "Population Movement and the Spread of HIV in Southern Africa." In *HIV/AIDS in South Africa*, edited by S. S. Abdool Karim and Q. Abdool Karim, 342–56. Cambridge: Cambridge University Press.

MacDonald, Raymond, Gunter Kreutz, and Laura Mitchell, eds. 2012. *Music, Health, and Wellbeing*. Oxford: Oxford University Press. https://doi.org/10.1093/acprof:oso/9780199586974.001.0001.

Mager, Anne Kelk. 2010. *Beer, Sociability, and Masculinity and South Africa*. Bloomington: Indiana University Press.

Maher, Lisa. 2002. "Don't Leave Us This Way: Ethnography and Injecting Drug Use in the Age of AIDS." *International Journal of Drug Policy* 13 (4): 311–25. https://doi.org/10.1016/s0955-3959(02)00118-4.

Mail and Guardian. 1998, March 6. *The Real Virodene Scandal*. Retrieved July 18 2024, from http://mg.co.za/article/1998-03-06-the-real-virodene-scandal.

Malloch, Stephen. 1999. "Mothers and Infants and Communicative Musicality." *Musicae Scientiae* 3 (1_suppl): 29–57. https://doi.org/10.1177/10298649000030s104.

Marler, Peter. 2000. "Origins of Music and Speech: Insights from Animals." In *The Origins of Music*, edited by Nils Wallin, Björn Merker, and Steven Brown, 31–48. Cambridge, MA: The MIT Press.

Martin, Dennis. 2013. S*ounding the Cape: Music, Identity and Politics in South Africa*. Sommerset West: African Minds.

Mattern, Mark. 1998. *Acting in Concert: Music, Community, and Political Action*. New Brunswick: Rutgers University Press.

Maultsby, Portia Katrenia. 2005. "Africanisms in African American Music." In *Africanisms in American Culture*, edited by Joseph Holloway, 326–55. Bloomington: Indiana University Press.

Mbali, Mandisa. 2013. *South African AIDS Activism and Global Health Politics*. Basingstoke: Palgrave Macmillan.

McConnell, Bonnie B. 2020. *Music, Health, and Power: Singing the Unsayable in the Gambia*. New York: Routledge.

McGrath, Joseph Edward, and Janice Kelly. 1986. *Time and Human Interaction: Toward a Social Psychology of Time*. New York: Guilford Press.

McGraw, Andrew. 2016. "Atmosphere as a Concept for Ethnomusicology: Comparing the Gamelatron and Gamelan." *Ethnomusicology* 60 (1): 125–47. https://doi.org/10.5406/ethnomusicology.60.1.0125.

McNeill, Fraser. 2011. *AIDS, Politics, and Music in South Africa*. Cambridge: Cambridge University Press.

Meintjes, Louise. 2003. *Sound of Africa!: Making Music Zulu in a South African Studio*. Durham: Duke University Press Books.

Meintjes, Louise. 2004. "Shoot the Sergeant, Shatter the Mountain: The Production of Masculinity in Zulu Ngoma Song and Dance in Post-Apartheid South Africa." *Ethnomusicology Forum* 13 (2): 173–201. https://doi.org/10.1080/1741191042000286185.

Merriam, Alan Parkhurst. 1964. *The Anthropology of Music*. Evanston, IL: Northwestern University Press.

Meyer, Leonard. 1989. *Style and Music: Theory, History, and Ideology*. Chicago: The University of Chicago Press.

Michie, Laura, and Vangeli Gamede. 2013. "The Toyi-Toyi Was out Weapon: The Role of Music in the Struggle Against Apartheid in South Africa." In *Sounds of Resistance: The Role of Music in Multicultural Activism*, edited by Eunice Rojas and Lindsay Michie, 251–70. Vol. 1 London: Bloomsbury Academic.

Miller, Daniel. 1987. *Material Culture and Mass Consumption*. Oxford: Basil Blackwell.

Mithen, Steven. 2005. *The Singing Neanderthals: The Origins of Music, Language, Mind, and Body*. Cambridge, MA: Harvard University Press.

Monelle, Raymond. 2000. *The Sense of Music: Semiotic Essays*. Princeton: Princeton University Press.

Moraes, Michele, Patricia da Conceição Rocha Rabelo, Valéria Pinto, Washington Pires, Samuel Penna Wanner, Raphael Szawka, and Danusa Dias Soares. 2018. "Auditory Stimulation by Exposure to Melodic Music Increases Dopamine and Serotonin Activities in Rat Forebrain Areas Linked to Reward and Motor Control." *Neuroscience Letters* 673 (April): 73–78. https://doi.org/10.1016/j.neulet.2018.02.058.

Morrell, Robert. 2003. "Silence, Sexuality and HIV/AIDS in South African Schools." *The Australian Educational Researcher* 30 (1): 41–62. https://doi.org/10.1007/bf03216780.

Morris, Gay. 1989. "Theatrical Possibilities of the Traditional Xhosa IINTSOMI: What Do They Offer Here and Now?" *South African Theatre Journal* 3 (2): 91–100. https://doi.org/10.1080/10137548.1989.9687980.

Mswela, Maureen. 2009. "Cultural Practices and HIV in South Africa: A Legal Perspective." *Potchefstroom Electronic Law Journal/Potchefstroomse Elektroniese Regsblad* 12 (4). https://doi.org/10.4314/pelj.v12i4.50053.

Muller, Carol Ann. 2008. *Focus: Music of South Africa*. 2nd ed. New York: Routledge.

Mybrugh, J. 2009. "In the Beginning There Was Virodene." In *The Virus, Vitamins and Vegetables: The South African HIV/AIDS Mystery*, edited by Kerry Culinen and Anso Thom, 1–15. Johannesburg: Jacana Media.

Nagasaka, Yasuo, Zenas C. Chao, Naomi Hasegawa, Tomonori Notoya, and Naotaka Fujii. 2013. "Spontaneous Synchronization of Arm Motion between Japanese Macaques." *Scientific Reports* 3 (1). https://doi.org/10.1038/srep01151.

Narsiah, Sagie. 2002. "Neoliberalism and Privatisation in South Africa." *GeoJournal* 57 (1–2): 3–13. https://doi.org/10.1023/a:1026022903276.

Nattrass, Nicoli. 2012. *The AIDS Conspiracy: Science Fights Back*. New York: Columbia University Press.

Neethling, Stephen Johan. 1990. "The Good, the Bad and the Ugly in Xhosa Iintsomi." *South African Journal of African Languages* 10 (4): 319–23. https://doi.org/10.1080/02572117.1990.10586863.

Nessler, Jeff, and Sara Gilliland. 2009. "Interpersonal Synchronization during Side by Side Treadmill Walking Is Influenced by Leg Length Differential and Altered Sensory Feedback." *Human Movement Science* 28 (6): 772–85. https://doi.org/10.1016/j.humov.2009.04.007.

Nessler, Jeff, David McMillan, Michael Schoulten, Teresa Shallow, Brianna Stewart, and Charles De Leone. 2013. "Side by Side Treadmill Walking with Intentionally Desynchronized Gait." *Annals of Biomedical Engineering* 41 (8): 1680–91. https://doi.org/10.1007/s10439-012-0657-6.

Nettl, Bruno. 2000. "An Ethnomusicologist Contemplates Universals in Musical Sound and Musical Culture." In *The Origins of Music*, edited by Nils Wallin, Björn Merker, and Steven Brown, 463–72. Cambridge: MIT Press.

Nettl, Bruno. 2015. *The Study of Ethnomusicology: Thirty-Three Discussions*. Urbana: University of Illinois Press.

Nickel, Patricia Mooney. 2012. "Philanthromentality: Celebrity Parables as Technologies of Transfer." *Celebrity Studies* 3 (2): 164–82. https://doi.org/10.1080/19392397.2012.679447.

Niehaus, Isak. 2005. "Masculine Domination in Sexual Violence: Interpreting Accounts of Three Cases of Rape in the South African Lowveld." In *Men Behaving Differently: South African Men since 1994*, edited by Graeme Reid and Liz Walker, 65–83. Cape Town: Double Storey Books.

Nilsson, Ulrica. 2009. "Soothing Music Can Increase Oxytocin Levels during Bed Rest after Open-heart Surgery: A Randomised Control Trial." *Journal of Clinical Nursing* 18 (15): 2153–61. https://doi.org/10.1111/j.1365-2702.2008.02718.x.

Nkoala, Sisanda Mcimeli. 2013. "Songs That Shaped the Struggle: A Rhetorical Analysis of South African Struggle Songs." *African Yearbook of Rhetoric* 4 (1): 51–61.

Okigbo, Austin. 2011. "Siphithemba – We Give Hope: Song and Resilience in a South African Zulu HIV/AIDS Struggle." In *The Culture of AIDS in Africa: Hope and Healing through Music*, edited by Gregory Barz and Judah Cohen, 285–98. Oxford: Oxford University Press.

Okigbo, Austin. 2014. "Music and the Politics of Culture in a South African Zulu HIV/AIDS Experience: Implications for 'Post-Apartheid.'" In *Contemporary Africa: Challenges and Opportunities*, edited by Toyin Falola, and Emmanuel Mbah, 175–90. New York: Palgrave MacMillan.

Okigbo, Austin. 2016. *Music, Culture, and the Politics of Health: Ethnography of a South African AIDS Choir*. Lanham, MD: Lexington Books.

Okigbo, Austin, and Bellarmine Ezumah. 2017. "Media Health Images of Africa and the Politics of Representation: A South African AIDS Choir Counter-Narrative." *Journal of Asian and African Studies* 52 (5): 705–21. https://doi.org/10.1177/0021909615608208.

Okpewho, Isidore. 1992. *African Oral Literature: Backgrounds, Character, and Continuity*. Bloomington, IN: Indiana University Press.

Okyere-Manu, B. 2013. "The Sexual Abuse of the Girl-Child in Pietermaritzburg, South Africa: Rethinking the Christian Response." In *Justice Not Silence: Churches Facing Sexual and Gender-Based Violence,* edited by E. Chitando and S. Chirongoma, 35–46. Stellenbosch: SUN Press.

Olaveson, Tim. 2001. "Collective Effervescence and Communitas: Processual Models of Ritual and Society in Emile Durkheim and Victor Turner." *Dialectical Anthropology* 26 (2): 89–124. https://doi.org/10.1023/a:1020447706406.

O'Leary, Ann, May Kennedy, Katina Pappas–DeLuca, Marlene Nkete, Vicki Beck, and Christine Galavotti. 2007. "Association between Exposure to an HIV Story Line in the Bold and the Beautiful and HIV–Related Stigma in Botswana." *AIDS Education and Prevention* 19 (3): 209–17. https://doi.org/10.1521/aeap.2007.19.3.209.

Olsen, Kathryn. 2014. *Music and Social Change in South Africa: Maskanda Past and Present*. Philadelphia: Temple University Press.

Oosthuizen, Gerhardus Cornelius. 1968. *Post-Christianity in Africa*. Grand Rapids, MI: William B. Eerdmans Publishing Company.

Overy, Katie, and Istvan Molnar-Szakacs. 2009. "Being Together in Time: Musical Experience and the Mirror Neuron System." *Music Perception* 26 (5): 489–504. https://doi.org/10.1525/mp.2009.26.5.489.

Pagel, Mark. 2017. "Q&A: What Is Human Language, When Did It Evolve and Why Should We Care?" *BMC Biology* 15 (1). https://doi.org/10.1186/s12915-017-0405-3.

Panksepp, Jaak. 2009. "The Emotional Antecedents to the Evolution of Music and Language." *Musicae Scientiae* 13 (2_suppl): 229–59. https://doi.org/10.1177/1029864909013002111.

Paulus, Paul. 2015. *Psychology of Group Influence*. 2nd ed. London: Taylor & Francis.

Pavlicevic, Mercédès, and Gary Ansdell, eds. 2004. *Community Music Therapy*. London: J. Kingsley Publishers.

Peltzer, Karl, Allan Davids, and Peter Njuho. 2011. "Alcohol Use and Problem Drinking in South Africa: Findings from a National Population-Based Survey." *African Journal of Psychiatry* 14 (1): 30–37. https://doi.org/10.4314/ajpsy.v14i1.65466.

Peltzer, Karl, and Shandir Ramlagan. 2011. "Perceived Stigma among Patients Receiving Antiretroviral Therapy: A Prospective Study in KwaZulu-Natal, South Africa." *AIDS Care* 23 (1): 60–8. https://doi.org/10.1080/09540121.2010.498864.

Pépin, Jacques. 2021. *The Origins of AIDS*. 2nd ed. Cambridge: Cambridge University Press.

Pickering, William Stuart Frederick. 2001. *Emile Durkheim: Critical Assessments of Leading Sociologists*. London: Routledge.

Pink, Sarah. 2006. *The Future of Visual Anthropology: Engaging the Senses*. New York: Taylor & Francis.

Pinker, Steven. 1997. *How the Mind Works*. London: Penguin Books.

Plato. 1980. "Republic." In *Plato the Collected Dialogues*, edited by Edith Hamilton and Huntington Cairns, 10th ed., 575–844. Princeton, NJ: Princeton University Press.

Posel, Dorrit. 2008. "AIDS." In *New South African Keywords*, edited by N. Sheperd and S. Robins, 13–24. Athens: Ohio University Press.

Powers, Theodore. 2020. *Sustaining Life: AIDS Activism in South Africa*. Philadelphia: University of Pennsylvania Press.

Poznik, David, Brenna Henn, Muh-Ching Yee, Elzbieta Sliwerska, Ghia Euskirchen, Alice Anne Lin, Michael Snyder, et al. 2013. "Sequencing y Chromosomes Resolves Discrepancy in Time to Common Ancestor of Males versus Females." *Science* 341 (6145): 562–65. https://doi.org/10.1126/science.1237619.

Ravignani, Andrea, Tania Delgado, and Simon Kirby. 2017. "Musical Evolution in the Lab Exhibits Rhythmic Universals." *Nature Human Behavior* 1, 0007. https://doi.org/10.1038/s41562-016-0007

Ray, Eileen Berlin, and Lewis Donohew. 1990. *Communication and Health: Systems and Applications*. Hoboken: Taylor and Francis.

Reed, Daniel. 2011. "'C'est Le Wake Up! Africa': Two Case Studies of HIV/AIDS Edutainment Campaigns in Francophone Africa." In *The Culture of AIDS in Africa: Hope and Healing through Music*, edited by Gregory Barz and Judah Cohen, 180–92. Oxford: Oxford University Press.

Reid, Graeme and Liz Walker. 2005. *Men Behaving Differently: South African Men since 1994*. Cape Town: Double Storey.

Riedel, Friedlind. 2020. "Atmospheric Relations: Theorising Music and Sound as Atmosphere." In *Music as Atmosphere: Collective Feelings and Affective Sounds*, edited by Friedlind Riedel and Juha Torvinen, 1st ed., 1–42. New York: Routledge.

Robins, Steven. 2005. "Introduction." In *Limits to Liberation after Apartheid: Citizenship, Governance, and Culture*, edited by Steven Robins, 1–28. Cape Town: David Philip Publishers.

Robins, Steven. 2004. "'Long Live Zackie, Long Live': AIDS Activism, Science and Citizenship after Apartheid." *Journal of Southern African Studies* 30 (3): 651–72. https://doi.org/10.1080/0305707042000254146.

Robins, Steven. 2008. *From Revolution to Rights in South Africa: Social Movements, NGOs, and Popular Politics after Apartheid*. Pietermaritzburg: University of KwaZulu-Natal Press.

Roenneberg, Till, and Martha Merrow. 2007. "Entrainment of the Human Circadian Clock." *Cold Spring Harbor Symposia on Quantitative Biology* 72 (1): 293–99. https://doi.org/10.1101/sqb.2007.72.043.

Rojek, Chris. 2012. *Fame Attack the Inflation of Celebrity and Its Consequences*. London: Bloomsbury Academic.

Ross, Robert. 1999. *A Concise History of South Africa*. Cambridge: Cambridge University Press.

Rousseau, Jean-Jacques. [1781] 1986. *Essay on the Origin of Languages*. Translated by Alexander Gode and John H. Moran. Chicago: University of Chicago Press.

Roy, William. 2010. *Reds, Whites, and Blues: Social Movements, Folk Music, and Race in the United States*. Princeton, CT: Princeton University Press.

Satgar, Vishwas. 2012. "Beyond Marikana: The Post-Apartheid South African State." *Africa Spectrum* 47 (2–3): 33–62. https://doi.org/10.1177/000203971204702-303.

Schechner, Richard. 2004. *Performance Theory*. London: Routledge.

Schneider, Hannah. 1998. "The Politics Behind Aids: The Case of South Africa. Politics Behind AIDS Policies." *Presentation to the 12th World AIDS Conference*. Geneva. June 28-July 3.

Schulkin, Jay, and Greta Bielaczyc Raglan. 2014. "The Evolution of Music and Human Social Capability." *Frontiers in Neuroscience* 8 (September). https://doi.org/10.3389/fnins.2014.00292.

Schumann, Anne. 2008. "The Beat That Beat Apartheid: The Role of Music in the Resistance against Apartheid in South Africa." *Stichproben – Vienna Journal of African Studies* 8 (14): 17–39.

Schütz, Alfred. 1951. "Making Music Together: A Study in Social Relationship." *Social Research* 18 (1): 76–97. https://www.jstor.org/stable/40969255.

Scott, James. 1990. *Domination and the Arts of Resistance: Hidden Transcripts*. New Haven: Yale University Press.

Seeger, Anthony. 1987. *Why Suyá Sing: A Musical Anthropology of an Amazonian People*. Urbana: University of Illinois Press.

Segatti, Aurelia, and Loren Brett Landau. 2011. *Contemporary Migration to South Africa: A Regional Development Issue*. Washington, D.C: World Bank.

Seltzer, Leslie, Toni Ziegler, and Seth David Pollak. 2010. "Social Vocalizations Can Release Oxytocin in Humans." *Proceedings. Biological Sciences* 277 (1694): 2661–6. https://doi.org/10.1098/rspb.2010.0567.

Shilling, Chris, and Philip Mellor. 1998. "Durkheim, Morality and Modernity: Collective Effervescence, Homo Duplex and the Sources of Moral Action." *The British Journal of Sociology* 49 (2): 193–209. https://doi.org/10.2307/591309.

Shilling, Chris, and Philip Mellor. 2001. *The Sociological Ambition: Elementary Forms of Social and Moral Life*. London: SAGE Publications Ltd.

Shisana, Olive, Thomas Rehle, Leickness Chisamu Simbayi, Khangelani Zuma, Sean Jooste, Nompumelelo Zungu, Demetre Labadarios, and Dorina Onoya. 2014. *South African National HIV Prevalence, Incidence and Behaviour Survey 2012*. Cape Town: HSRC Press. http://hdl.handle.net/20.500.11910/2490.

Sidahmed, Abdel Salam, Walter Soderlund, and Donald Briggs. 2010. *The Responsibility to Protect in Darfur: The Role of Mass Media*. Lanham, MD: Lexington Books.

Singhal, Arvind, and Everett Rogers. 2004. "The Status of Entertainment-Education Worldwide." In *Entertainment-Education and Social Change: History, Research, and Practice*, edited by Arvind Singhal, Michael John Cody, Everett Rogers, and Miguel Sabido, 3–20. Lawrence Erlbaum Associates Publishers.

Singhal, Arvind, and Everett Rogers. 2012. *Entertainment-Education: A Communication Strategy for Social Change*. London: Routledge.

Sirayi, Mzo. 2012. *South African Drama and Theatre from Pre-Colonial Times to the 1990s: An Alternative Reading*. Bloomington: Xlibris Corporation.

Sithole, Nkosinathi. 2014. "Beyond African Nationalism: Isaiah Shembe's Hymns and African Literature." *Literator* 35 (1). https://doi.org/10.4102/lit.v35i1.1069.

Sloboda, John. 2010. "Music in Everyday Life: The Role of Emotions." In *Handbook of Music and Emotion*, edited by Patrik Juslin and John Sloboda, 493–514. Oxford: Oxford University Press.

Small, Christopher. 1987. *Music of the Common Tongue: Survival and Celebration in Afro-American Music*. London: Calder Publications.

Small, Christopher. 1998. *Musicking: The Meanings of Performing and Listening*. Middletown, CT: Wesleyan University Press.

Soares, Ana Maria, and Maher Georges Elmashhara. 2020. *Emotional, Sensory, and Social Dimensions of Consumer Buying Behavior*. Hershey, PA: IGI Global, Business Science Reference.

Somers, John William. 2008. "Interactive Theatre: Drama as Social Intervention." *Music and Arts in Action* 1 (1): 61–86. https://www.musicandartsinaction.net/index.php/maia/article/view/interactivetheatre

Sontag, Susan. 2013. *Illness as Metaphor and Aids and Its Metaphors*. New York: Penguin Books.

Steindl, Christina, Eva Jonas, Sandra Sittenthaler, Eva Traut-Mattausch, and Jeff Greenberg. 2015. "Understanding Psychological Reactance: New Developments and Findings." *Zeitschrift Für Psychologie* 223 (4): 205–14. https://doi.org/10.1027/2151-2604/a000222.

Stephan, Klaus Martin, Michael Thaut, Gilbert Wunderlich, Wilfried Schicks, Bozhi Tian, Lutz Tellmann, Thomas Schmitz, et al. 2002. "Conscious and Subconscious Sensorimotor Synchronization—Prefrontal Cortex and the Influence of Awareness." *NeuroImage* 15 (2): 345–52. https://doi.org/10.1006/nimg.2001.0929.

Stewart, Donald, and Yoon Irons. 2018. "Music, Public Health, and Health Promotion: Can Music Be a Social Determinant of Health?" In *Music, Health and Wellbeing: Exploring Music for Health Equity and Social Justice*, edited by Naomi Sunderland, Natalie Lewandowski, and Dan Bendrups, 17–31. London: Palgrave Macmillan. https://doi.org/10.1057/978-1-349-95284-7_2.

Stige, Brynjulf, and Leif Edvard Aarø. 2011. *Invitation to Community Music Therapy*. London: Taylor & Francis.

Stige, Brynjulf, Gary Ansdell, Cochavit Elefant, and Mercédès Pavlicevic. 2010. *Where Music Helps: Community Music Therapy in Action and Reflection*. Farnham and Burlington, VT: Ashgate.

Stone, Mollie Spector. 2015. "Black South African Choral Music and the Struggle against HIV." Unpublished PhD thesis, Northwestern University.

Styns, Frederik, Leon van Noorden, Dirk Moelants, and Marc Leman. 2007. "Walking on Music." *Human Movement Science* 26 (5): 769–85. https://doi.org/10.1016/j.humov.2007.07.007.

Sutoo, Den'etsu, and Kayo Akiyama. 2004. "Music Improves Dopaminergic Neurotransmission: Demonstration Based on the Effect of Music on Blood Pressure Regulation." *Brain Research* 1016 (2): 255–62. https://doi.org/10.1016/j.brainres.2004.05.018.

Switzer, Les. 1997. *South Africa's Alternative Press: Voices of Protest and Resistance, 1880–1960*. Cambridge: Cambridge University Press.

Tausig, Ben. 2019. *Bangkok Is Ringing: Sound, Protest, and Constraint*. Oxford: Oxford University Press.

Taylor, Timothy Dean. 2012. *The Sounds of Capitalism: Advertising, Music, and the Conquest of Culture*. Chicago: The University of Chicago Press.

Taylor, Timothy Dean. 2016. *Music and Capitalism: A History of the Present*. Chicago: The University of Chicago Press.

Terrier, Philippe, Vincent Turner, and Yves Schutz. 2005. "GPS Analysis of Human Locomotion: Further Evidence for Long-Range Correlations in Stride-to-Stride Fluctuations of Gait Parameters." *Human Movement Science* 24 (1): 97–115. https://doi.org/10.1016/j.humov.2005.03.002.

Terry, Peter, Costas Karageorghis, Michelle Curran, Olwenn Viviane Martin, and Renée Parsons-Smith. 2020. "Effects of Music in Exercise and Sport: A Meta-

Analytic Review." *Psychological Bulletin* 146 (2): 91–117. https://doi.org/10.1037/bul0000216.

Thaut, Michael, Gerald Curtis McIntosh, and Volker Hoemberg. 2015. "Neurobiological Foundations of Neurologic Music Therapy: Rhythmic Entrainment and the Motor System." *Frontiers in Psychology* 5 (February). https://doi.org/10.3389/fpsyg.2014.01185.

Thompson, Leonard Monteath. 2001. *A History of South Africa*. 3rd ed. New Haven: Yale University Press.

Treichler, Paula. 1987. "AIDS, Homophobia and Biomedical Discourse: An Epidemic of Signification." *Cultural Studies* 1 (3): 263–305. https://doi.org/10.1080/09502388700490221.

Tufte, Thomas. 2005. "Entertainment-Education in Development Communication: Between Marketing Behaviours and Empowering People." In *Media and Glocal Change: Rethinking Communication for Development*, edited by Oscar Hemer and Thomas Tufte, 159–74. Buenos Aires: Glaxco.

Tufte, Thomas. 2008. "Fighting AIDS with Edutainment: Building on the Soul City Experience in South Africa." In *Communication for Development and Social Change*, edited by Jan Servaes, 327–46. London: Sage.

Turino, Thomas. 2008. *Music as Social Life: The Politics of Participation*. Chicago: The University of Chicago Press.

Turner, Victor. 1969. *The Ritual Process: Structure and Anti-Structure*. New Brunswick: Aldine Transaction Publishers.

van Buren, Kathleen. 2011. "Music, HIV/AIDS and Social Change in Nairobi, Kenya." In *The Culture of AIDS in Africa: Hope and Healing Through Music and the Arts*, edited by Gregory Barz and Judah Cohen, 70–84. Oxford: Oxford University Press.

van der Berg, Servaas. 2006. "Public Spending and the Poor since the Transition to Democracy." In *Poverty and Policy in Post-Apartheid South Africa*, edited by Haroon Bhorat, and Ravi Kanbur, 201–31. Cape Town: HSRC Press.

Vernallis, Carol. 2004. *Experiencing Music Video: Aesthetics and Cultural Context*. New York: Columbia University Press.

Visser, Maretha, and Heather Sipsma. 2013. "The Experience of HIV-Related Stigma in South Africa." In *Stigma, Discrimination and Living with HIV/AIDS: A Cross Cultural Perspective*, edited by Pranee Liamputtong, 205–28. Dordrecht, Netherlands: Springer Netherlands.

von Lieres, Bettina. 2005. "Culture and the Limits of Liberalism: Marginalisation and Citizenship in Post-Apartheid South Africa." In *Limits to Liberation after Apartheid: Citizenship, Governance, and Culture*, edited by Steven L Robins, 22–56. Cape Town: David Philip Publishers.

von Scheve, Christian. 2012. "Collective Emotions in Rituals: Elicitation, Transmission, and a 'Matthew Effect.'" In *Emotions in Rituals and Performances*, edited by Axel Michaels and Christopher Wolf. London: Routledge.

Waldmeir, Patti. 1998. *Anatomy of a Miracle: The End of Apartheid and the Birth of the New South Africa*. New Brunswick, N.J: Rutgers University Press.

Walker, Gavin Robert. 2018. "'Our Songs Were Our Stones': Song and Struggle in the Treatment Action Campaign." *Journal of Contemporary African Studies* 36 (2): 175–90. https://doi.org/10.1080/02589001.2018.1464130.

Walker, Gavin Robert. 2019. "Music Research in a South African Higher Education Institution." *Action, Criticism, and Theory for Music Education* 18 (3): 144–71. https://doi.org/10.22176/act18.3.144.

Walker, Gavin Robert. 2021a. "Sexual Diversity and Local Values in a Rural South African University Town." *Gender and Education* 34 (4): 379–93. https://doi.org/10.1080/09540253.2021.1960279.

Walker, Gavin Robert. 2021b. "'A Song Is Not Just a Song': Community Mobilisation and Psychosocial Healing in South Africa's Aids Crisis." *African Studies* 80 (3–4): 310–34. https://doi.org/10.1080/00020184.2021.1975532.

Walker, Gavin Robert. 2022a. "Emotive Media as a Counterbalance to AIDS Messaging Fatigue in South Africa: Responses to an HIV/AIDS Awareness Music Video." *AIDS Education and Prevention* 34 (1): 17–32. https://doi.org/10.1521/aeap.2022.34.1.17.

Walker, Gavin Robert. 2022b. "Analysing Behavioural Outcome Effectiveness in a Musical Theatre-Based HIV/AIDS Intervention among South African Farm Workers." *Health Promotion International* 37 (5). https://doi.org/10.1093/heapro/daac146.

Walker, Gavin Robert. 2022c. "Pulsing Bodies and Embodying Pulse: Musical Effervescence in a South African Community Outreach Programme." Anthropology & Medicine 29 (3): 289–304. https://doi.org/10.1080/13648470.2021.1994335

Walker, Gavin Robert. 2024. "Musicking in Applied Theatre: Exploring Interdisciplinary Approaches to Drama-Based Health and Social Interventions." *Research in Drama Education: The Journal of Applied Theatre and Performance* 29 (1): 187–205. https://doi.org/10.1080/13569783.2023.2249409.

Werner, Craig Hansen. 2006. *A Change Is Gonna Come: Music, Race & the Soul of America*. 2nd ed. Ann Arbor, MI: University of Michigan Press.

West-Eberhard, Mary Jane. 2003. *Developmental Plasticity and Evolution*. Oxford: Oxford University Press.

Wetherell, Margaret. 2012. *Affect and Emotion: A New Social Science Understanding*. Los Angeles: Sage.

Wildenthal, Lora. 2013. "Humanitarianism in Postcolonial Contexts: Some West European Examples from the 1960s to the 1980s." In *Colonialism and Beyond: Race and Migration from a Postcolonial Perspective*, edited by Eva Bischoff and Elisabeth Engel, 104–23. Berlin: LIT Verlag Münster.

Wilson, Margaret, and Peter Cook. 2016. "Rhythmic Entrainment: Why Humans Want to, Fireflies Can't Help It, Pet Birds Try, and Sea Lions Have to Be Bribed."

Psychonomic Bulletin & Review 23 (6): 1647–59. https://doi.org/10.3758/s13423-016-1013-x.

Winkler, István, Gábor Péter Háden, Olivia Ladinig, István Sziller, and Henkjan Honing. 2009. "Newborn Infants Detect the Beat in Music." *Proceedings of the National Academy of Sciences* 106 (7): 2468–71. https://doi.org/10.1073/pnas.0809035106.

Yoshida, Itsuko, Toshio Kobayashi, Sabitri Sapkota, and Kongsap Akkhavong. 2013. "A Scale to Evaluate Music for Health Promotion in Lao PDR: Initial Development and Assessment." *Arts & Health* 5 (2): 120–31. https://doi.org/10.1080/17533015.2012.736395.

Yurdum, Lidya, Manvir Singh, Luke Glowacki, Thomas Vardy, Quentin Atkinson, Courtney Hilton, Disa Sauter, Max Krasnow, and Samuel Mehr. 2023. "Universal Interpretations of Vocal Music." *Proceedings of the National Academy of Sciences* 120 (37): e2218593120. https://doi.org/10.1073/pnas.2218593120.

Zimbardo, Philip. 2008. *The Lucifer Effect: Understanding How Good People Turn Evil.* New York: Random House.

Zivotofsky, Ari, and Jeffrey Hausdorff. 2007. "The Sensory Feedback Mechanisms Enabling Couples to Walk Synchronously: An Initial Investigation." *Journal of NeuroEngineering and Rehabilitation* 4 (1): 564–70. https://doi.org/10.1186/1743-0003-4-28.

Zuch, Melanie, and Mark Lurie. 2012. "'A Virus and Nothing Else': The Effect of Art on HIV-Related Stigma in Rural South Africa." *AIDS and Behavior* 16 (3): 564–70. https://doi.org/10.1007/s10461-011-0089-6.

Index

About the Author

Gavin Robert Walker is an ethnomusicologist and associate professor at Minjiang University. Prior to this, he held the Andrew W. Mellon postdoctoral research fellowship at the Africa Open Institute at Stellenbosch University. He received his PhD in ethnomusicology from the School of Oriental and African Studies (SOAS), University of London, and an MA in musicology from Durham University. Gavin's research focuses on the performing arts in health and social interventions, advocacy, and well-being. His work has appeared in academic journals including *Health Promotion International*, *Anthropology & Medicine*, *African Studies*, *Gender and Education*, *AIDS Education and Prevention*, and the *African Journal of AIDS Research*.

www.ingramcontent.com/pod-product-compliance
Lightning Source LLC
LaVergne TN
LVHW010304020626
840297LV00003B/38